PRAISE FOR *WITH SPRINKLES ON TOP*

"*With Sprinkles on Top* is an essential read for partners who are having trouble connecting because they have different fantasies and desires. Stefani Goerlich weaves together research, clinical insight, and practical tips in an accessible and affirming style. Readers will walk away with the tools they need to explore their sexuality and cultivate more satisfying intimate relationships."

JUSTIN J. LEHMILLER, PhD
host of the *Sex and Psychology Podcast*, author of *Tell Me What You Want*

"At a time where kink is becoming more mainstream, this text should be in the hands of everyone who is in kink, kink aware, or kink adjacent. Stefani Goerlich's tactful offering is easily digestible and will help readers feel more informed, more understood, and more reflective of the person they are and who they want to become. *With Sprinkles on Top* is an excellent resource with compelling content that will be relevant for many years to come. Goerlich's expertise and brilliance shines vividly as a well-respected clinician in this field."

MARLA RENEE STEWART
sexologist

"*With Sprinkles on Top* is for everyone who has ever wondered if they, or their partner, was a pervert. Most of us have sexual desires we're afraid to share for fear of rejection. Goerlich's newest book offers concerned readers the most important possible message: 'You're ordinary.' Even those of us with diverse sexual interests are, at the end of the day, ordinary people. Along the way, you'll learn critical skills and techniques on how to ethically and responsibly integrate your honest sexual desires into your relationship with respect, dignity, and mutuality."

DAVID J. LEY, PhD
author of *Ethical Porn for Dicks*

"This book is far more than the average BDSM how-to! *With Sprinkles on Top* is an invaluable resource for couples nervous about kink but eager to explore the intimacy and trust it brings. With a disarming and empathetic approach, Stefani Goerlich guides readers through custom-crafting intentional, mutually fulfilling erotic experiences while challenging bias and shame with compassion. Packed with science-backed facts, exercises, and real-world vignettes, Goerlich reframes kink for what it truly is: joyous play, adventurous self-exploration, and a path to deep connection. Whether you're looking to add a little spice or navigate the complexities of coming out as kinky to a vanilla partner, this transformative guide provides the tools you need to move forward with authenticity and curiosity."

SUNNY MEGATRON
sexologist, host of the Showtime Original series *Sex with Sunny Megatron*

"*With Sprinkles on Top* is a must-read—in fact, a positive game changer—for anyone in a couple in which one partner identifies as kinky and the other as vanilla or simply uncertain if kink is for them. This engaging and easy-to-read book, full of relatable quotes and stories, is based in both science and the clinical wisdom of one of the most experienced sex therapists in the field. Throughout the book, Dr. Goerlich's genuine compassion shines through as she guides readers to a deeper understanding of themselves and their partners. *With Sprinkles on Top* is a road map that will lead kinky people and their vanilla partners to be more understanding of one another and closer than ever before."

LAURIE MINTZ, PhD
author of *A Tired Woman's Guide to Passionate Sex* and *Becoming Cliterate*

"You scream, I scream, we all scream for . . . Stefani Goerlich! She shows us that 'being vanilla' isn't boring and bland, it's sexy and exciting! *With Sprinkles on Top* is the best book on understanding and navigating the world of kink that I've ever read."

IAN KERNER, PhD, LMFT
New York Times bestselling author of *She Comes First*

with sprinkles on top

Also by Stefani Goerlich, PhD

The Leather Couch: Clinical Practice with Kinky Clients

*Kink-Affirming Practice: Culturally Competent Therapy
from the Leather Chair*

with sprinkles on top

Everything Vanilla People
and Their Kinky Partners
Need to Know to Communicate,
Explore, and Connect

STEFANI GOERLICH, PhD

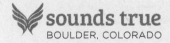

sounds true
BOULDER, COLORADO

Sounds True
Boulder, CO

This book is not intended as a substitute for the medical recommendations of physicians, mental
health professionals, or other health-care providers. Rather, it is intended to offer information to
help the reader cooperate with physicians, mental health professionals, and health-care providers
in a mutual quest for optimal well-being. We advise readers to carefully review and understand
the ideas presented and to seek the advice of a qualified professional before attempting to use
them. Some names and identifying details have been changed to protect the privacy of individuals.

Published 2023

Cover design by Charli Barnes
Book design by Meredith Jarrett
Illustrations © 2023 Natsu/Cry_Tm

Printed in the United States of America

BK06578

Library of Congress Cataloging-in-Publication Data
Names: Goerlich, Stefani, author.
Title: With sprinkles on top : everything vanilla people and their kinky partners need to know to
    communicate, explore, and connect / Stefani Goerlich, PhD.
Description: Boulder, CO : Sounds True, 2023. | Includes bibliographical references and index.
Identifiers: LCCN 2022058939 (print) | LCCN 2022058940 (ebook) | ISBN 9781649630346
    (paperback) | ISBN 9781649630353 (ebook)
Subjects: LCSH: Bondage (Sexual behavior) | Sexual excitement. | Sex.
Classification: LCC HQ79 .G644 2023 (print) | LCC HQ79 (ebook) |
    DDC 306.77/5--dc23/eng/20230111
LC record available at https://lccn.loc.gov/2022058939
LC ebook record available at https://lccn.loc.gov/2022058940

10 9 8 7 6 5 4 3 2 1

To the Nachos, my pocket-buddies
And to Wolf, my bashert

Contents

The worksheets in this book are available to download and print at stefanigoerlich.com/with-sprinkles-on-top-worksheets.html#/.

INTRODUCTION

I Promise, I'm Not a Pervert

When I first sat down to write this book, I kept getting caught up with the question of punctuation—specifically, quotation marks. Beginning our time together with a bold, declarative statement that "I promise, I'm not a pervert" might make you think that I sound rather defensive. After all, there is a strong possibility that someone close to you has uttered this same sentence fairly recently. And there's an equally strong possibility that you're not entirely confident that you believe them. If so, you have likely picked up this book looking for reassurance, information, perhaps even some guidance; and the last thing I want to do is sound defensive.

This is especially true because so many of the folks who come to my office seeking therapy begin their first session with these same words. "I promise," they tell me, "I'm not a pervert." Sometimes I am told, "I'm afraid my partner is some kind of pervert." When these conversations happen, I ask the person sitting across from me what the word *pervert* means to them. Their answers are remarkably consistent. They tell me that they are *not* a:

"Creepy guy lurking in the bushes."

"Predator."

"Weirdo into messed-up sex."

"Child molester."

"Freak."

"Sinner."

"Some broken creature with fucked-up fantasies."

1

And you know what? I have never met someone who meets the criteria for perversion that they describe when I ask. So who are these people who find themselves in my office talking about their secret fantasies and sexual behaviors? The ones who can tell me oh-so-easily what they are not? They are . . . ordinary.

My clients are college kids and business executives, attorneys and auto mechanics, clergy and kindergarten teachers, and everything in between. Which makes sense because kinky people, to quote Wednesday Addams, "look just like everyone else." The media tends to portray kinky folks in one of two ways: dangerous predators (*Body of Evidence*, *American Horror Story*) or the butt of jokes (*Bonding*, *Exit to Eden*). Very rarely are kinky people portrayed as happy, healthy people with well-rounded lives and fulfilling relationships. And this stereotype is not only unfair but also incorrect.

That's not to say that there aren't some traits that BDSM practitioners have in common. In general, kinksters tend to be white, well educated, and affluent.[1] (Which is not to say that you have to be any of these things to thrive as a kinky person! Kinky people exist in all forms and places and are valid and welcome in the BDSM community.) Their mental health is the same as that of the general population. Multiple studies show that kinky people tend to be just as mentally healthy as their vanilla peers. Along the same lines, they are no more likely to commit a crime than a nonkinky person. By almost every metric, kinky people truly are "just like everyone else." In fact, surveys show that somewhere between 2 to 8 percent of people identify as kinky. That means that BDSM practitioners are about as common as redheads or people who are left-handed.

In 2018, I conducted an unofficial survey of just over two hundred BDSM community members.[2] The majority of those who responded were female—with women outnumbering men two to one. The majority (51 percent) held college degrees, which is significantly higher than the general population, and 37 percent held jobs in management or professional services such as medicine or law. Half of them identified as monogamous in their relationships, while another 21 percent said they preferred a polyamorous dynamic with their partners. (Polyamory is one form of consensually nonmonogamous relationship.) Twenty-two percent of surveyed kinksters described themselves as "spiritual but not religious," while 14 percent identified as Christian.

One of the most fascinating things that I learned while doing this survey was the frequency with which the respondents liked to engage in BDSM. Half told me that they like to engage in kinky play every week or every few weeks. Roughly one in four said that they tried to include elements of BDSM into their everyday life. This took different forms for different folks. For some respondents, giving their partner a spanking every few weeks was all they needed to feel happy and sexually fulfilled. Others told me that they were kinky every day because they called their partner "Ma'am" or had a set of relationship rituals that they enacted together daily. For the people who shared their lives with me, the most important element was the relationship they had with their partners. For them, BDSM is always relational but only sometimes sexual.

And really, that's why you're here. Numbers and data are nice to know, but the reason you picked up this book is because you're worried about what these differences between you and your partner mean for your relationship. You might be afraid that your partner is dangerous. You might be afraid your partner won't accept you. More likely, you're afraid that one or both of you are just plain weird. And not weird in the wearing-quirky-glasses-and-taking-up-the-banjo way, but weird in a way that indicates some kind of fundamental flaw you failed to notice in the beginning. There are many ways that the kinky elephant in the room may have been revealed. Best-case scenario, it came up during a direct conversation. Maybe the kinkier person sat their partner down and said that there was something they'd held secret that they now wanted to share in the relationship. Maybe the knowledge came to the vanilla person when they stumbled across an email, an open browser tab, or an illicit text message. If knowledge of our partner's kinky nature is accompanied by deception or infidelity, the pain is compounded exponentially. But it is important, for our conversation, to separate the two discoveries. Being kinky is not an excuse for infidelity. But fear of revealing our kinky interests often results in secrecy. In fact, 50 percent of kinksters say that they are afraid of how their partner might react to their interest in BDSM.[3] Fear breeds secrecy, and secret-keeping can feel very much like betrayal. If these words feel familiar to you, it's time to bring BDSM out of the shadows.

WHAT ARE BDSM AND KINK, ANYWAY?

Throughout this book, you're going to see me use the terms *BDSM* and *kink*—sometimes interchangeably. Heck, we've already started! So it probably makes sense to take a minute to define these terms for you. **Kink** is an umbrella term that simply means "anything that falls outside of the sexual, erotic, or relational norm." That's a pretty big umbrella! And it means different things in different places. In America, for example, heterosexual monogamy is the statistical norm. In America, we might consider it kinky to have multiple spouses or to be married without being sexually exclusive with our spouse. In other parts of the world, however, those choices are *not* the norm and so would not be seen as "kinky." On the other hand, **vanilla** is a term used to describe all that is normative (as in "what the largest number of people do") within a given place or culture. That's why you'll hear many sex therapists say, "Normal is just a setting on the dryer."

A **fetish** is a sexual attraction to an object or body part that is not usually seen as sexual. Again, that "usually seen" piece means that fetishes are also culturally specific. In some parts of the world, it is considered criminally indecent to see a woman's hair, for example. Hair, in those cultures, is sexualized and considered an erotic attribute in a way that it is not in America or other parts of the world. Here, we might see someone who gets turned on when they see high-heeled shoes, who fantasizes about sex with a partner wearing high heels, or who perhaps even needs their partner to be wearing high heels in order to be turned on and sustain their arousal. Shoes in our culture are not typically seen as sexual objects, so that would be considered a form of fetish. There are many who consider BDSM to be a kind of fetish. The assumption is that this kind of intimacy is rooted in desire and arousal. And sure, it can be! But BDSM can also be a relationship style, and there exist many BDSM practitioners who incorporate elements of BDSM into their lives without any sexual contact at all. If this all sounds complicated or confusing, I understand. Let's take a closer look.

We often think about BDSM as a single thing: a universe built out of leather, metal, rubber, and rope inhabited by only two kinds of people—demanding, egotistical sadists and their groveling, pathetic slaves. The reality is that *BDSM* is an umbrella term composed of three smaller abbreviations—each of which carries distinct meaning and can be explored in isolation or in a myriad of combinations, depending on the desires and boundaries of those involved. **Bondage and discipline** are best described as an exchange of *control*. **Dominance and submission**, on the other hand, are an exchange of *authority*. **Sadism and masochism** often sound like the scariest of the three, but at its core, SM is all about the giving and receiving of *sensation*. Let's take a look at each of them in greater depth.

Bondage is often identified as many kinky people's point of entry into BDSM. They recall childhood experiences of wearing toy handcuffs while playing cops and robbers or being tied up during a vigorous game of pirates, and they realize that their reactions to these experiences went a bit beyond what others might have felt. Bondage, at its most basic, is the practice of using rope, ties, cuffs, or other tools to restrict movement. In a study of adults, 4.8 percent of women and 4.1 percent of men say that they have either tied up their partner or have been tied up as a part of sex.[4] The sensations of being restrained—the squeeze of the rope, the challenge of maintaining a specific position, or the tension in their muscles as they do so—feels quite pleasurable to many; and they enjoy incorporating these feelings into their sexual interactions—or even their relaxation habits, similar to the way others might use a weighted blanket.

Discipline in BDSM is also about control. But rather than controlling movement, this discipline is about exercising control over behavior—sometimes during role-play scenarios (teacher and naughty student, for example) and sometimes in everyday life. This often takes the form of observing mutually-agreed-upon rules that apply to one or more person(s) in the relationship. These rules are put in place to strengthen and enhance the relationship between the rule maker and the rule follower. Discipline, in this case, is often realized through the self-discipline of the rule follower to consistently abide by a structured routine. Likewise, there are often consequences when the rule follower fails to follow the routine, which often takes the form of discipline from or as directed by the rule maker. For example, in 2017, 20 percent of women and 14.2 percent of men told researchers that they had been spanked as a part of sex.[5] However, that doesn't mean that all discipline needs to be physical! A couple might agree that the rule follower will bring the rule maker a cup of coffee in bed each morning. If the rule follower forgets one morning, the rule maker might require them to write "I will bring my spouse a coffee in bed each morning without fail" one hundred times. Both developing the habit of making the coffee and the willingness to write the lines when they forget are acts of discipline.

Dominance and submission occurs when one person (the submissive) agrees to cede some of their personal authority to another (the dominant), an arrangement typically abbreviated as D/s. D/s takes many forms, from very modest (perhaps a wife agrees to let her husband select her panties each morning) to what is known as "total power exchange," where the submissive partner defers to their dominant in every area of their life. Often D/s and discipline blend together, with rules and structure built into the exchange of authority; but it is quite possible to only practice D/s. Perhaps this means that partners agree to maintain a "traditional" home with a male head of household and his supportive wife, taking on clearly defined roles and tasks based on gender. Alternately, D/s can look like a female dominant who takes over decision-making authority across the board; she gives her submissive partner a weekly allowance and a set of assigned tasks, and maintains a strict hierarchy between herself and her partner. D/s in one form or another is the most common form of BDSM, often including elements of the other practices, but primarily centered around the roles of decision maker and decision follower. In one study exploring BDSM relationships, 41.1 percent of participants identified as submissive (or a variation of the term), 28.2 percent as dominant (or some variation), and 22.5 percent as switch—someone who enjoys taking on both roles at different times or with different people.[6]

Why do people choose to cede authority to another person? Why would someone want to take authority over their partner? There are as many answers to these questions as there are kinky people on Earth, but there is a persistent theme that tends to shine through: it relaxes them. There are many folks in this world who feel most comfortable and confident when they have a degree of influence over their environment. They like being the person with the answers, calling the shots, and influencing those around them. On the other hand, there are people who find giving up this task just as relaxing. They enjoy shrugging off the day-to-day responsibilities that they must carry and just let someone else be the one to call the shots for a time. When these two kinds of people find each other, it often results in a relationship that feels easy, supportive, comforting, and safe.

Then there is a group of people who might leave the casual bystander feeling distinctly unsafe: those who call themselves sadists. The idea that there are people—our friends, neighbors, coworkers—who enjoy inflicting pain on others can be discomfiting. And that reaction makes sense when we think about where we usually hear about sadistic people! We usually encounter the terms *sadist* or *sadistic* in the context of horror movies or *Law & Order* episodes, and it often evokes images of serial killers and movie monsters. In her memoir *Sex with Shakespeare*, about life as a spanking fetishist, Jillian Keenan observes that "coming to terms with the details of our sexual identities is hard for everyone. . . . This process is often even more difficult for sadists. I can't imagine how scary and confusing it must be to realize, in the early stages of sexual development, that you long to 'hurt' the people you desire."[7] The fear that they will harm us results in a great deal of stigma toward folks who enjoy sadistic play. This fear is based in part on the stereotypes of the malignant sadist that we see on screens. It is reinforced by the fact that both sadism and masochism continue to be included as disordered behavior within the fifth edition of the *Diagnostic and Statistical Manual of Mental Disorders* (DSM-5), the guidebook used by mental health providers to identify and diagnose mental illnesses.

The inclusion of these labels within the DSM-5 is controversial. Many sex therapists believe that they should be removed because there is a clear difference between the kinky person who enjoys making their consenting partner wiggle and gasp and the malignant person who actively seeks to cause lasting harm to people who do not ask for their attention. For our purposes, the important things to know are that the criteria for calling sadism a mental health disorder is carefully written to exclude consensual BDSM and that kinky sadism is more common than we might realize. Approximately 3 percent of women and 7.5 percent of men identify as sadists and enjoy giving their partner a variety of intense sensations and observing their reactions—the winces and gasps, the writhing, and the moans.[8] Watching their partner as they process and move through the physical experiences that they create for them is a sensory delight to the sadist. And sure, for many people these sensations feel like pain. But pain is a very subjective thing, and even when giving their partner painful sensations, the goal of the kinky sadist is never to cause them harm. They simply want to savor the deep trust, intimate connection, and sensory symphony of inflicting intense sensation on a willing partner who enjoys a bit of temporary suffering.

Where sadists are feared, masochists are often pitied. We assume that they must be broken, traumatized, or otherwise dysfunctional. This is a flawed stereotype based on our own limited understanding. After all, we usually try to avoid pain, don't we? So isn't it logical to think that there must be something wrong with those who seek it out instead? Perhaps. Yet research shows us that masochists are no more likely to have a history of trauma or mental illness than the general population. So what's the deal? Why do 24 percent of women and 14 percent of men enjoy taking pain as a part of their sexual play?[9] The elegant, counterintuitive answer is "because it feels good." Receiving pain causes the body to release endorphins. Endorphins not only inhibit the brain's ability to receive pain signals but they also increase the sensation of pleasure.[10] In the same way that adding sea salt to a caramel magnifies its sweetness, so too does a bit of pain enhance our experience of pleasure. And it's not just the physical that sees a boost; sadomasochistic play has been shown to evoke a measurable increase in the relationship closeness reported by partners afterward.[11]

This is not to say that masochists enjoy any and every kind of pain. Just because there are painful sensations they enjoy in one setting does not mean that they enjoy experiencing pain in any setting, as there is also "bad pain." Bad pain might mean a dental cavity or the results of a broken arm or even a particularly bad bout of stomach flu, and research indicates that even the most hardened masochist does not enjoy a migraine.[12] Good pain is often experienced after a hard workout or during childbirth. The hallmark of good pain is the notion that it is constructive rather than destructive. A constructive outcome to masochistic play might be a sense of pride and strength in being able to endure a challenging experience. It might be the strong bond and sense of connection a masochist feels with their partner afterward. It can also be as simple as the pleasure they receive from the rush of endorphins. Masochism in this form is not a type of self-harm. The DSM-5 makes a clear distinction between consensual sexual sensory exchange (even intense sensations that we might call painful) and a desire to purge oneself of deep emotional distress through self-injury. Masochism in consensual kink is not an expression of depression or distress. Rather, it is a powerful, multisensory quest that takes the masochist deep into their awareness of their own physicality before bringing them back again into a space of connection and partnership with the sadist who facilitated the journey and kept watch over the physical and emotional safety of their masochistic partner during this scene.

The theme in each of these BDSM practices is that of relationship. Kinky people enjoy BDSM because it feels good, sure. But more importantly, it helps them build stronger, closer relationships. This includes the relationship that they have with their own body, which can be incredibly powerful in a world where we are bombarded with messages telling us we'll never quite be young, sexy, or fit enough. It is also about the relationship they have with their partners—the deep trust that comes from being willing to take or give control even just for a while; the feelings of peace and support experienced when both partners know who has the authority in a given moment or situation; and the physiological bond that is created when giving and receiving intense sensations. The goal of BDSM is never to harm (although admittedly sometimes it might hurt a bit) either partner. BDSM is about creating intentional, cocreated, deeply fulfilling, physical, emotional, and sometimes sexual bonds between people.

MEET YOUR FRIENDLY NEIGHBORHOOD SEX THERAPIST

But why on earth should you take my word for it? Most likely I have never met you or your partner. Why should my opinion carry any weight at all when you are trying to wrap your head around the knowledge that your partner enjoys the sights, sounds, and perhaps experiences of something you might find mildly off-putting, confusing, degrading, or even completely abhorrent? Who am I to offer reassurances without any direct knowledge of your specific situation? Perhaps it's time I introduced myself:

Hi, I'm Stefani. And I promise, I'm not a pervert.

When I started my career in social work twentyish years ago, while I was studying to earn my bachelor's degree, I began as a first response survivor advocate. In this role, I carried a pager (yes, I am carried-a-pager-years-old!) and was on call for one twenty-four-hour shift per week. If the pager went off, this meant that someone had been sexually assaulted and was being

brought to my agency for a forensic medical exam and, often, a police interview. It was my job to be present with this person (usually a woman, but
far too frequently a child) who had been raped within the last forty-eight
hours. I provided comfort, crisis intervention, and prophylactic medication
to reduce their risk of pregnancy or sexually transmitted illness. I sat with
them during the police interview and tried to protect them from hostile or
judgmental lines of inquiry. Sometimes I had to tell the parents of my child
survivors that we had placed a mandatory call to Child Protective Services
and that I would be present to support them during the interview that
would shortly follow—assuming they didn't hate me for having to make
the call in the first place. It was my job to bear witness to the suffering of the
survivors who came to us for help and to try to mitigate this suffering
where and when I could.

After graduation, I worked at an agency serving high-risk women and
girls in Detroit, Michigan. Many of my clients were commercial sex workers,
walking the streets of Michigan Avenue or dancing in clubs (with or without
the required "cabaret license"). Some were trafficking survivors, coerced into
sex work they never chose for themselves. Others were young teens, strug-
gling to stay safe while feeling trapped between an abusive homelife and the
unforgiving city streets. Once again, my role was crisis interventionist and
advocate. I gave out condoms and dental dams like candy, and provided
baby formula, winter coats, and prom dresses. I learned what the term *sur-
vival sex* meant, and I gained a deep appreciation for the strength of women
who, with nothing else to their names, chose to feed themselves and their
children by leveraging the only resource they had left—their bodies.

A few years after completing graduate school, I started my private therapy
practice, Bound Together Counseling. I had spent over a decade witnessing
what could happen when our sexuality and our physicality were weaponized against us. I had taken a little girl's Easter dress and placed it into an
evidence bag for the state police to collect. I had coordinated a multia-
gency plan to evacuate a sexually exploited young woman from her father's
home and move her to an undisclosed location. I had begged foster parents not to send away young children in their care who were acting out
after years of abuse. I had helped throw holiday parties for beloved clients
whom others derisively called "streetwalkers." I was and still am proud of

the work I have done for victims of domestic and sexual violence, but I was also tired. I wanted to flip the coin and help my clients reclaim their sexuality. I wanted to help people have happier, healthier relationships with their bodies, their partners, and themselves. So I decided to return to school and pursue certification as a sex therapist.

One of the steps in becoming a sex therapist is to complete a multiday learning experience called the Sexual Attitudes Reassessment (SAR). It is an intentionally challenging experience, designed to expose potential sex therapists to the full spectrum of human sexuality—both that which we find lovely and empowering and that which we often find repellant or even criminal. The purpose is to create a space for us to learn more about the myriad of ways in which humans express and explore their sexuality and to take time to reflect on our reactions to these expressions. It is a time to normalize some behaviors and to understand others. It is a space for us to sit with our own feelings and to recognize where our therapeutic limits, interests, and biases might be.

Sitting in the room with a group of people who were my peers (fellow therapists, nurses, sex educators, and ob-gyns), I listened as they sighed romantically at the video we watched of a couple in their eighties making gentle, careful love. I watched their faces as they confronted their own questions and presumptions around disabled bodies and sexuality. I helped brainstorm strategies to support the emotional health of men and women experiencing sexual dysfunction. Then came our hour-long presentation on BDSM and fetishes.

The mood in the room shifted. The reverence was gone. There were quiet jokes and not-so-subtle giggles. The audience's gaze shifted from respectful to something more akin to amusement. The people we were watching on screen, in their leather and chain, were not seen as potential clients so much as they were a midafternoon spectacle, something entertaining to break up the day. My heart broke and my hackles rose. To be fair, the SAR process had done exactly what it was intended to do; it had revealed a point of tension, discomfort, resistance, and misinformation within the audience around this particular community. I decided then and there that these people were my people, that I would strive to do for them what I had done for every person I'd ever sat beside as their sexuality and relationship choices were second-guessed, criticized, and shamed.

That moment gave me a gift. It let me witness firsthand the kind of passive stigma and benign aggression that so many kinky people experience. Since that day, I have spoken at conferences around the country on BDSM and kink-affirming practice. I have written two books intended to help mental health providers better understand and meet the needs of kinky people. I have written blogs for both Psychology Today and the PornHub Sexual Wellness Center, helping people unpack various alternative relationship styles and niche sexual interests. I have earned a PhD in clinical sexology, an emerging discipline that is on the cutting edge of sexuality research and treatment. And I have worked with so many kinky clients in my practice. I have dedicated my professional life to being a bridge builder between the margins and the mainstream. However, there was one aspect of that work that I had overlooked until more and more couples started seeking therapy with me: my clients' nonkinky partners.

The Kinky Client Comes Out

Discovering that one's partner is kinky can be scary. It raises a number of questions, many of which feel threatening to our relationship and our sense of self:

"How could someone enjoy something like this?"

"Does this mean they're gay/lesbian?"

"Is my partner dangerous?"

"Are they cheating on me?"

"Does this mean they're not attracted to me?"

"What else have they been keeping from me?"

"Did I ever know them at all?"

These questions twist in the mind, leaving us feeling discombobulated and adrift. Sometimes we wish we could go back in time, to the hours just before we stumbled across that website or sat down to have "a talk." Sometimes it feels easier to just not know and to pretend that everything is as it was before the revelation. The most important thing to hear right now is that, for all intents and purposes, everything is still as it was before. Your partner is still the person you fell in love with, still the person you built a life with, still the person you've enjoyed romance and passion with, still the person you've raised children with. The love between you remains constant. What has changed is your awareness of their curiosity, their creativity, their desire. And change is almost always scary—not just for the vanilla person wrestling with this new information but also for the kinky partner waiting with bated breath to see what happens next.

So where do we go from here, now that you know what you both know? That, my friend, is where I come in. As a certified sex therapist who specializes in teaching about and working with gender, sexuality, and relationship minorities, I am going to give you the information, suggestions, and support you need to make the decisions that feel right for you. The purpose of this book is *not* to convince you to become kinky or to engage in any activity that makes you feel uncomfortable or unsafe. Nor is it to tell you to repress your kinky urges. I am first and foremost an advocate, and my belief in the importance of bodily autonomy and informed consent are inviolable. That said, I am here to offer context and nuance to your understanding of BDSM, to demystify it where I can, to create space for you to consider what exploring some elements of your partner's interests might do for you as an individual and for your relationship, and to make sure you feel confident and supported in whatever decisions you choose to make.

SO, WHAT'S THE GAME PLAN?

We'll start this process by reflecting on how you and your partner might be feeling right now. Anger is a common reaction to revelations that have been held secret. Likewise, it's normal to feel ashamed, embarrassed, and afraid. We'll spend some time processing how you're feeling about learning about your partner's interests in kink . . . and also building some empathy for them. It's quite likely that as you sit here with me, trying to wrap your head around this new discovery, that they are also sitting with their own feelings of embarrassment and fear. From there, I'll give you some of the latest research on BDSM practices and practitioners: who they are and where they come from. We'll talk about fantasy versus reality and parse out abusive behavior from consensual kink. Once we've built an evidence-based framework for understanding BDSM, we'll explore some of the ways in which you can use this new information. That conversation will include a range of opportunities, from clarifying and setting boundaries for yourself to beginning an exploratory journey into some well-lit corners of the BDSM world. It's only after this point that we'll dive into the question of what "normal" means . . . and what it doesn't. This decision is intentional. I want you to come into this process with a delicious curiosity. I don't want you to limit your explorations and conversations to an arbitrary standard that may or may not feel right for you. Only after you've had these moments of discovery and definition will we take on the work of validating and "normalizing" your authentic self—no matter how kinky or vanilla that self might be. We'll talk about negotiating your relationship on your terms, which can be as creative or conservative as you want. Finally, we'll look at what happens if you get to the end of this conversation and realize that your ideal relationship dynamic is one that is completely free of BDSM in any form. The realization that the divide between ourselves and our partner might be insurmountable is devastating; if, at the end of our time together, that is where you stand, please know that I stand with you. My goal, of course, is not to end in that place. I genuinely believe that most relationships are capable of expanding to hold a wonderful variety of romantic expressions, ways of connecting, opportunities for exploration and play . . . the sprinkles on the sundae of our relationships.

In the *Journal of Couple & Relationship Therapy*, Amity Pierce Buxton identifies seven stages that we go through after discovering that our partner identifies as a sexual minority. These include:

1. Disorientation and disbelief (chapter 1)

2. Facing and acknowledging reality (chapter 2)

3. Accepting the new changes in the relationship (chapter 3)

4. Healing from the pain and stress caused by the disclosure (chapter 7)

5. Learning to refocus on ourselves and our identities (chapters 4 and 5)

6. Reconfiguring and refocusing on our belief systems and worldviews (chapter 6)

7. Transforming or moving on (chapter 8)[13]

We will explore each of these stages and how each of you may experience them, recognizing that there are no right answers and no definitive outcomes. We will emerge on the other side more informed, more insightful, and better prepared to make whatever decision is best for you and your partner.

Whenever we are encountering something new or difficult, it is helpful to find others who have navigated these waters already. The wisdom that comes from the lived experiences of others is invaluable. To that end, I've included short interviews with folks who have already encountered some of the relationship challenges and opportunities we'll be exploring together. These anonymized essays are the real, firsthand words of actual people (both vanilla and kinky) who volunteered to share their stories with me and, by extension, with you. Some of them are colleagues and acquaintances of mine. Some are clients being treated by my professional peers. Each of them took time to speak with me and share the lessons they've learned through their own relationship struggles and successes.

This book is a work of compassion and hope, sensuality and pragmatism. Together, we will gain appreciation for the full spectrum of sexual and relational diversity—including the fullness and depth of "vanilla" relationships. Not everything in this book will appeal to you. Some of the topics might be off-putting or even triggering to read about. That's okay! This book is not homework, and you're not being graded. Feel free to read the chapters out of order, to skim, to skip a paragraph or two. My only request is that if you do encounter content you simply cannot read, you debrief that reaction with your partner. I'm not here to cause you distress . . . but I encourage you to interrogate your discomfort, even as you respect the boundaries you discover together. Keep in mind that this book is one tool you can use to begin to bridge the differences between you and your partner. It is not a prescription. If you find things here that don't work for you, that's 100 percent okay. I highly recommend that you seek out a kink-affirming certified sex therapist in your area to work with as you read and consider the exercises and information I offer. Visit kapprofessionals.org and aasect.org to help you find someone practicing in your community.

One of my favorite expressions in the BDSM community is "Don't yuck their yum." Too often we rush to assume that "vanilla" somehow means bland, dull, or otherwise lacking. Many of my clients have sat across from me in my office and worried that they were too vanilla for their partners to appreciate. When this happens, I go to my bookshelf. There, amid the sexology guides and psychological tools, I keep something unusual: the tenth edition of the King Arthur Baking Company's *Essential Cookie Companion*. I hand this to them and encourage them to flip through the pages. I ask them to find a recipe that doesn't require vanilla. Rich, heady vanilla is the foundation in every delicious variation. You can't experience the diversity of either cookies or sex without first appreciating the nuance that vanilla contributes to the mix. Vanilla is worthy of celebration! And, sometimes, vanilla is worthy of adornment—not with a flavor that will alter or mar its intrinsic perfume but with a bit of decoration, a touch of flair . . . a dash of sprinkles on top.

Navigating Discovery and Disclosure

There's something sexy about a secret identity. We love watching James Bond's intellectual tango with a seductive (but dangerous) femme fatale. He knows she's working for the enemy . . . but does she know he knows? The tension between them is delicious. Likewise, we experience a vicarious triumph when the glass slipper slides onto Cinderella's foot and the impoverished scullery maid is revealed to be the belle of the ball. And every viewer's heart catches in their chest when Buttercup pushes the Dread Pirate Roberts down the hillside, only to hear him call out "As you wish!" The entire superhero genre is built on the theme of secret identities and dramatic life-changing revelations. But have you ever wondered how Bruce Wayne's girlfriend felt when she realized her billionaire boyfriend liked to put on a latex bodysuit and wander around the shadier side of town? Was she *really* cool with her partner role-playing as a flying rodent in front of all of Gotham's best and brightest? Sure, secret identities are sexy *hypothetically* . . . but maybe (just maybe) Mr. and Mrs. Smith would have had a happier, healthier marriage if they could have just told each other they were both assassins?

THE PROBLEM WITH SECRETS

This is not a book about infidelity. There are many great resources available on that topic, and I think it's important to let the experts on affairs do that work. This is a book about secrets—keeping them, revealing them, and discovering them, and the impact that secrecy can have on a relationship. These secrets can take many forms—from illicit encounters to private truths, spiritual fears, and personal longings. Whether these secrets have been held for a few days or a lifetime, discovering that our partner has been keeping secrets from us can feel akin to infidelity, especially when those secrets are connected to their sexuality. Discovering that they've been holding something back—another relationship, a hidden interest, information about their history—can challenge our understanding of who our partner is.

Not all secrets are bad, of course. We may not ever want our partner to know about our bimonthly appointments to get our upper lip waxed, for example. And planning an anniversary surprise is a delightful secret to keep. A desire for privacy is not the same as secret-keeping. Our partners have a right to lock their phones, for example, or to choose not to discuss their sexual fantasies with us if that makes them feel uncomfortable. Everyone is entitled to a private life. Privacy is what allows us to thrive and grow as individuals, separate and distinct from our partners. Privacy is a right that allows us to set and maintain healthy boundaries. Secrecy, on the other hand, can be a problem. Withholding information from our partners can create walls in the relationship that lead to isolation, distance, and resentment. Secrecy can feel protective for the one holding the secrets because it is often a product of fear, which can make disclosure feel like an insurmountable challenge.

Clinical sexologist Claudia Six, author of the book *Erotic Integrity*, explains that "people keep secrets for the same reason they lie. Because they don't think the truth will be accepted. It's called being deceitful by omission. People are afraid they'll be rejected, shamed, or made wrong, so they keep things secret. When we don't feel good about something, we don't want others to know, even if it's completely harmless."[1] When these truths come out, the realization that our partner is not the person we believed them to be (which is not the same as saying they are a *bad* person!) can leave us emotionally shaken. Likewise, when their secrets are revealed (either by choice or by accident), the secret-keeper is left feeling exposed and vulnerable—fearful emotional reactions just as strong as those of the person making the discovery. And yet when our emotions are running high, it can be terribly difficult to recognize that our partner might be feeling much the same way.

Confusion

Human beings are storytelling creatures. We crave order, predictability, and consistency; and we use narrative to make and create meaning from the world around us. When what we think we know is thrown into question, confusion is a natural response. Ten thousand years ago, we sat around campfires and told stories to explain why the rivers rose above their banks or didn't, why the crops thrived or failed, why two people fell in love or passed each other by. Today we better understand the natural world. But other people, and their behavior and choices, are just as obtuse to us today as they were to our ancestors.

From the fairy-tale stories of frogs turned to princes and epic quests to discover secret names, to the ever-evolving origin stories of power and personality found in the worlds of DC Comics and Marvel, to the first time Anastasia Steele ever sets foot in Christian Grey's red room in E. L. James's *Fifty Shades of Grey*—we continue to create mythologies for one another (and ourselves) that help us understand who people are and why they do the things they do.

When we learn a new piece of information we didn't have before, our brains struggle to find a context that makes sense. Sometimes this is easy: "Oh, I never knew that you'd considered joining the Peace Corps, but I can totally see you doing something like that! Tell me more about what led you to change your mind!" Other times, however, we learn something that challenges the story we tell about ourselves and the people in our world in a way that is disruptive and confusing. We can't move forward cognitively or emotionally until we've made sense of this new information.

Imagine you've been working on a jigsaw puzzle. Five hundred pieces, slowly building an image of the Eiffel Tower. You place the final piece, completing the picture, but as you go to move the box out of the way so that you can photograph your completed project, you hear a rattle. Five more pieces fall out. They're sparkly silver holograms—they make no sense in the context of your Parisian vista. And what's more? You've already *finished* the puzzle!

You were certain that you knew the story of your puzzle journey: purchasing this particular scene; carefully sorting the edge pieces, then parsing out the various colors into piles of umber, beige, green, yellow, red—no sparkly silver bits anywhere; working for an hour or so each evening to fit the pieces together, slowly watching it all take shape. Taking each step, until the final moment you went to capture your success, and then . . . Those five extra pieces confused everything. It's not that you think the puzzle is wrong. The picture is complete; there are no gaps left to fill. It's just that now you know it's going to bother you until you figure out where those five sparkling pieces came from.

You check your collection. Maybe you have a puzzle with a hologram design that got mixed with this one. You call the manufacturer—perhaps this was the result of a factory error they need to address. You look online. Could it be that these are pieces to a bonus puzzle you can collect if you purchase more from the same maker? The new pieces don't diminish the view of Paris that you have created. They just lack context. So? In our effort to make sense of the confusion, we create meaning and context through storycrafting. To *make them* make sense for us. To resolve the inevitable discomfort that confusion causes. While I've worked with couples who are navigating the realization that one partner *isn't* as kinky as they might have originally let on, the majority of couples who come to me are processing the reverse—the discovery that one partner has kink fantasies and desires that they have not previously shared.

Whether you have learned of your partner's interests in BDSM and kink by stumbling across a surprising link in their browser history, by discovering a cache of toys and tools hidden in the back of the closet, or because they sat you down and gently, thoughtfully shared this aspect of themselves with you, it's quite likely that you feel confused. When we learn that our partner is aroused by something that we're not, particularly something we find offensive or off-putting, it can be confusing. We don't understand how this kind, intelligent, sexy human that we know so well can be into . . . that (whatever that is), and our instinctive response—our very human response—is to create a story that gives context to this new information. Unfortunately, because of the anger that can precede confusion, the tales we craft for ourselves are often quite unkind both to ourselves and to our kinky partner. This is because, for many of us, the story that makes the most sense at first is a tale of betrayal.

Betrayal

When we learn that our partners are aroused by that which we are not, particularly if this interest has been kept secret or deliberately withheld from us, it can leave us feeling as if we don't know them at all. We worry that this secret interest says something about them as a person, a partner, and perhaps even as a parent. The more we ruminate, the faster the confusion evolves and shifts into indignation: How *dare* they keep this from us!? How could they *want* this? *Do* this? *Be* this? We have a right to know what kind of creepy/dirty/gross/perverted/weird/scary stuff they were into before we ever agreed to spend the rest of our lives with them! Something that, admittedly, had never impacted our daily lives or relationship before this knowledge came to light suddenly seems to have tainted every aspect. In the absence of informed consent, our minds create stories of betrayal.

At the same time, our partners have had their innermost desires laid bare to us. Perhaps by choice, but possibly not. They are exposed, vulnerable, likely fearful of the embarrassment and judgment they are bracing for from the person they love most in this world. *Their* anger at having their privacy violated or their secrets laid bare, *their* confusion about why someone who loves them so much is reacting to them with such distress and distance, make sense now too. After all, this is just one facet of them, one small piece of the person that we love so much. It has not mattered before. They struggle to understand why this knowledge might change the nature of the relationship now. "I am still who I've always been," they say to us. "You just know me a little better, a little deeper, now." Our reactions, no matter how understandable, can feel like betrayal to them too.

Guilt and Shame

For many of us, both kinky and not, guilt and shame make up the gooey center of our response to conversations about kinks, fetishes, and identity. While we use these terms interchangeably, they aren't actually the same thing. We feel guilty for our behaviors. We feel shame about who we are.[2] When we learn that our partner is kinky, it is easy to mistake one for the other and assume that because we are wrestling with our own feelings of distaste that they must likewise feel ashamed of their interest in BDSM. And many do. Unfortunately there is still a great deal of stigma surrounding society's understanding of BDSM. It's sadly all too common for kinky people to internalize this stigma and use social norms as a measure of personal value. They feel broken, dirty, unworthy, even evil; the shame that some kinky folks carry is unfair and does them tremendous harm. We're going to examine this in more depth in chapter 2. Thankfully, however, not all kinky people feel ashamed of their interest in BDSM. We have come a long way culturally in our understanding and portrayals of gender, sexuality, and relationship differences. While there's still a long way to go, there is a growing understanding that BDSM and fetishes can play a healthy role in the lives of healthy people and can be enjoyed without shame. The more significant challenge for the couples I encounter in my practice isn't shame but guilt.

When we learn that our partner is kinky, either directly from them or in any other way, guilt is their most common initial response. Guilt at having caused us hurt, confusion, anger, or pain. Guilt at having held a secret from us. Guilt for having engaged in behaviors that we might have preferred they not. Guilt for breaking promises or even vows. Guilt for not being the person we thought they were. While it may not be true in every situation, for many of the couples who find themselves in my office, it is the *behaviors* that have damaged the relationship. This is a crucial piece for us to understand: who they are has not changed (although we may get to know them better, deeper, and more completely moving forward); what they have *done* may have caused us pain. That pain—the notion that someone we've loved so deeply and trusted so completely might do something that could hurt us—can make us fearful.

FEAR AND LOATHING IN THE BEDROOM

Fear is both an emotion and a physical experience. When our brain is activated by something scary, it is unable to differentiate between types of dangers. Whether we've noticed a tiger lurking in the darkness outside of our primal cave or an OnlyFans charge on our twenty-first-century credit card statement, the brain reacts the same. So, before we talk about what we might be fearful of now that the secrets have come out, let's talk a bit about how our body responds to those fears. Understanding what is experience and what is emotion is a key piece of working through the fears evoked by this new information.

Neuroception is the process by which our autonomic nervous system (the brain and nerves) takes in information from the environment, our body, and others around us to form a steady subconscious stream of lightning-fast risk assessments. "When people metaphorically speak about having a 'bullshit meter' or a 'gut instinct,' they're often referring to a complex neural circuitry that signals a neurophysiological process that allows us to either relax when oriented to safety or engage in survival-mode strategies when oriented to a perceived threat."[3] This gut instinct is often activated when we are concerned about secret-keeping in our relationships, and we respond to these feelings physiologically as well as emotionally.

When our brain senses danger, it signals our body to release the stress hormones cortisol and adrenaline. These chemicals signal our heart to beat faster, our lungs to breathe stronger, and our blood to flow toward our limbs, preparing them to run away and evoking that pins-and-needles sensation we associate with being afraid. These rapid physical changes affect other things too: our field of vision changes,[4] our ability to form memories is impaired, and the parts of our brain that control emotional regulation, understanding others' body language, and rational decision-making shut down temporarily.[5] Needless to say, none of this is conducive to actually working through our fears effectively with our partners, especially at a time when we might be looking at them as the source of our distress! So, let's unpack some of those fears.

Broken Vows

When one secret is revealed, it's quite logical to worry that there are others we haven't discovered yet. For many of us who find out our partner has sexual interests and desires that we were unaware of, infidelity can be a primary concern. This can be especially true of (but certainly not limited to) folks in traditionally monogamous relationships. We're afraid that if our partner is aroused by something that we've never done (or perhaps never even heard of), they must have done it somewhere with someone else. While it makes sense to connect dots in this manner, what we understand about the connection between fantasy and cheating is that it isn't always quite that straightforward.

I spoke to Eric Anderson, a psychologist and sociologist who has published over a hundred scholarly articles and twenty-five books on topics related to masculinity, sexuality, and sports. Among these is *The Monogamy Gap: Men, Love, and the Reality of Cheating*.[6] Anderson was also the former chief science officer for a famous infidelity dating website. He describes cheating as a form of wish fulfillment—often carnal wishes for men, more romantic wishes for women. And while it is true that we often conflate wishes with fantasies, there are many things that people fantasize about all the time that they have no intention of acting out in real life, though Anderson points out that we often channel these fantasies into socially acceptable outlets: "Fantasy is mostly just fantasy. It remains fantasy in coz play, in video games about war, in movies and porn."[7] From fantasy football leagues to Renaissance festivals, we act out our own wish fulfillment in dozens of ways.

And it seems that what many kinky people wish for most is simply acceptance. When surveyed by KinkD.com, a BDSM dating site, the majority of respondents who admitted to stepping outside of their committed relationship in order to pursue a BDSM dynamic did so primarily because of isolation and frustration. Thirty-two percent of unfaithful kinksters said that they cheated on their partners due to "fear of talking about BDSM desires," while 26 percent were motivated by "failure in introducing BDSM into [their] relationship/marriage."[8] These feelings of loneliness and rejection led to more fantasy-driven motivators, such as "searching for a new sense of self" (17 percent) or "the seductive nature of the transgression" (13 percent).[9] This lines up with Anderson's findings. He explains that when we want things, whether it's a hot quickie with the Uber driver or a heavy flogging scene, and we can't have them, we often come to "view (our) partners as the obstacle to that. This creates animosity, even if subtly."[10] And when we start to feel hostile toward our partners? Particularly when we feel rejected or alone? It can motivate us to seek out validation, connection, and comfort elsewhere.

Sex isn't the only way to meet those needs. The debate around emotional infidelity occurs daily, if not hourly, in couples therapy sessions around the world. The line between friendship and something that may feel more threatening varies from person to person and is often defined according to standards that are measured as much by gut instinct as rational mind. Social, religious, cultural, and psychological factors all come into play when trying to determine when (or if) an external friendship has become *too much* and is now a threat to the couple. This is particularly true when kink-identified folks who are unable to explore BDSM within their relationship form friendships with others who share their interests outside of the relationship.

Researchers who study emotional infidelity often describe it as "sharing or exchanging personal and sensitive information with others who are not spouses, emotionally distancing from his/her partner . . . absent (or missing) from joint activities, loss of sexual desire and interest in discussing the future together."[11] It is quite possible for a kinky person in a mixed BDSM/vanilla relationship to form healthy, supportive relationships with other kinky people that do not result in the distance and emotional separation described here. This is possible primarily when they are able to share these relationships with their partners. As we have seen from Anderson's work, secrecy fosters separation, separation can cultivate resentment, and resentment blooms into detachment. Where we create space for our kinky partners to have friendships with other kinky people, and we bring these friendships (if not their conversation topics or activities) into our relationships, the motivation for emotional infidelity decreases significantly. In chapter 7 we'll look at some ways this can work.

One other form of infidelity that brings many couples (and not just kinky/vanilla couples) to therapy is financial infidelity. Researchers at Indiana University have defined financial infidelity as "engaging in any financial behavior that is expected to be disapproved of by one's romantic partner and intentionally failing to disclose this behavior to them."[12] One of these researchers, Jenny Olson, states that "financial infidelity has the potential to be as harmful for relationship health and longevity as sexual infidelity."[13]

Financial secrecy can be a serious problem in mixed kinky/vanilla relationships because often paid resources such as membership websites, erotic content creators, or professional BDSM practitioners are the kinky partner's only outlet for exploring their interests. This can create a pattern of purchasing and concealment that can quickly spiral out of control for the person making the purchases. We see similar behavior patterns in folks who shop online and then hide the purchases from their spouse or who gamble and conceal their losses with "creative" household accounting. In fact, many times it has been a financial discovery that has brought a mixed-desire couple to my office for the first time; and the double whammy of financial deception combined with secret-holding around sexual desire can be incredibly difficult for the discovering partner to process. In fact, the way my kinky clients budget and pay for their BDSM interests is a key element in our safety planning process together!

Risky Business

So far, many of the concerns that we've addressed have focused on the ways in which our partner's kinks might affect us and our relationship with them. But it's also true that many vanilla people come to counseling because they are worried about their *partner's* health and safety. There are so many myths and misconceptions surrounding what it means to be kinky or to engage in BDSM that it's not uncommon for kinky people to be met not with hostility or anger from their vanilla partners but with deep worry for their physical, mental, and emotional well-being. This genuine concern comes from a place of love, but for the kinky person, it can feel like a form of rejection.

We're going to take a deeper look at who kinky people are, what their BDSM interests mean, and what the research tells us about kinky personality types in chapter 2. But I want to take a moment here to address the worry about risk that so many of my vanilla clients have expressed for their kinky partners. The BDSM community places a strong emphasis on consent. In fact, its consent culture is such that the kink community may actually have lower rates of domestic violence and sexual assault than the general population.[14] A natural extension of the prominence that consent carries as a value within the world of BDSM is a strong framework for risk assessment. After all, someone must be fully aware of the risks of any activity before they can properly consent to it! The BDSM community understands that everyone's personal risk profile is different, and what might feel quite safe for one person (posting nude photos online, for example) might feel quite risky to another. That's why the community has developed a variety of models to help one another assess risk and make informed choices based on their own unique circumstances. The most popular of these include:

Safe, Sane, and Consensual: The oldest and possibly original community risk framework first came in the 1980s. It was first proposed by Mark Berkenwald, Bob Gillespie, and David Stein of the New York Gay Male S-M Activists (GMSMA) and remained popular until the early 2000s when mental health advocates within the BDSM community pointed out that using "sane" to indicate safety was causing harm to kinksters living with mental health concerns.[15] While you'll still hear it used as a shorthand slang for "safe play," it's mostly been replaced by the concept of RACK.

Risk-Aware Consensual Kink: In a world where 1.35 million people die in car accidents every year[16] and another twenty people annually are killed by cows,[17] RACK starts with an acknowledgment that very little in life is truly safe. Instead, the priority here is on educating yourself to know what the risks are and how to mitigate them . . . and then making sure that everyone involved understands exactly what they're agreeing to do (or avoid doing). We know that driving is riskier than touring the petting zoo, and we make our choices accordingly. And if our spouse or partner would rather walk to the zoo than ride with us? We respect their right to set personal limits around their own risk levels. That's the consent piece.

The Four C's—Caring, Communication, Consent, and Caution: The newest BDSM risk framework, introduced in 2014 in a paper published by a team of researchers at Idaho State University,[18] the Four C's model takes RACK and expands it to emphasize the importance of communication with and caring for one's partner. Whether this is someone the kinky person is partnering with for a single BDSM scene[19] or for a lifetime, the Four C's says that they have an obligation to understand not only what their partner wants and needs during the scene itself but who they are as people—their culture and identity, the nature of their relationships (with each other and with others), what they value, and how they express these values so that each interaction is a model of safety, trust, and respect.

One of the most supportive things that a vanilla person can do for their kinky partner is to talk to them about their personal risk framework. Instead of operating from a place of media-driven fears of rash decision-making and dangerous behaviors, asking them to share which of these frameworks they prefer and how they apply it to their own BDSM interests and pursuits can be a wonderfully affirming way to begin to explore your partner's kink interests together. Especially if you don't feel ready to begin learning more about the specific details of their erotic desires, starting from a place of "Tell me how you make decisions about what to watch/attend/access/respond to" can feel like a safe starting point. Being able to develop your own personal risk framework and communicate your boundaries to your partner is a vital part of the journey you're taking together. Why not start by asking them, with genuine curiosity and without any attempt to influence their choices, how they make these decisions for themselves?

Heaven and Hell

Some of my favorite couple-clients are young newlyweds raised in deeply religious homes who got married because it was the only way to do what they wanted to do without worrying about eternal damnation. They come to me in their early twenties, often lacking much in the way of general sex-ed knowledge, and it becomes my work—my pleasure, actually—to help them figure out how all of this sex stuff works, now that they're finally allowed to try it out. I teach them about anatomy, foreplay, communication. I help to normalize intimacy and increase their comfort levels with each other, with their bodies, and with themselves. But there is one question I'm asked quite frequently that I don't have an answer to: "Isn't that a sin?"

For many of the couples that I work with, religious traditions and the beliefs they've been raised with are an important part of their personal identities and family life. They cannot, nor do they wish to, separate their values from their relationship, and so reconciling the latter with the former becomes an important part of our work in counseling.[20] I love working with religious clients because as a person of faith myself, I believe wholeheartedly that sex and intimacy are divine gifts created to offer us a uniquely human way to express love and give pleasure to those we care about. Most religious traditions offer some version of this idea within their teachings.[21] Though, admittedly, a few don't. Finding space within my client's existing belief system (after all, it's never my job to try to change their mind) for them to embrace who they are, who their partner is, and what they desire individually and for each other can be some of the most challenging and rewarding work we do together.

The judicial code tells us what is legal. Philosophy offers guidance about what is ethical. Only you can decide what is moral—based on your own personally held values and beliefs. Whole books—indeed, entire disciplines—have been created to address the vast topic of sexual and relational morality. It's far more than what we can cover together here. I think it's important to acknowledge the role that religion and spirituality can play in this conversation for many and to recognize that this book can't answer those questions. I do believe that there is space for "yes" within most religious traditions, and I will offer a few quotes along the way to inspire you as we venture onward and deeper into this conversation. I'd encourage you to honor the values and traditions that you bring to this journey, to consider some of the resources offered at the end of this chapter, and to proceed through the rest of this book accompanied and informed by those beliefs.

Navigating Discovery

I found out early in our relationship that my husband had watched trans porn when he was younger, and I had read it was somewhat common for straight(ish) men, so I worked through it. I was on his phone, trying to send myself family photos, and I saw a screenshot of a sex shop order. I went upstairs to look for the stuff and it was right there in his drawer. I discovered sex toys (dildos, plugs) and subsequently looked at his internet history, which I know was wrong, but I wanted to know.

I felt like my life was falling apart, honestly. I gave myself about a day to think about it, so I wouldn't come in angry, and then I confronted him about what I'd found. It took him a while to be honest, but he's not a very good liar, so I was able to pull things out. He was pretty open, and a couple days later we set aside time to be alone, talk, and explore. My one caveat was that I could ask him anything I wanted, and he had to be honest. He agreed.

It took a while for me to trust him, and I still don't totally. He said that he'd always enjoyed trans porn and had gone down a rabbit hole into a sissification fetish—where people are forced into being more feminine as part of someone dominating him—over the years. The desire to be a sissy is new to him, but once I found out and asked him to open up to me about everything, he expressed more of an interest in moving from just watching trans porn to doing more together.

At first I was worried that he was trans, because he was clearly aroused by it. But it's more of a cross-dressing and humiliation kink for him. It made me totally uncomfortable. I would do it again on a special occasion for him, but it's not super comfortable for me. Kink plays a large role now. We incorporate mild feminization, pegging, and dirty talk. We also send photos and try to explore some of our shared interests. He says that he doesn't do much on his own because he's able to "live his fantasy" now. I'm sure that's not entirely true.

It's difficult. I think I struggle because it brings sexuality and gender identity questions. I wish he understood my need to discuss the kinks. Understandably, he doesn't want to be constantly questioned, but I have difficulty trusting him after he kept secrets from me for a very long time. I obsess about it. I'll google, which is a bad idea. I read too much into a picture or a text. You feel uneasy when your partner has kept secrets from you. When it's something that's not you or not something you do together, it feels like you're being cheated on. That's how it felt to me—like I was being lied to and cheated on. I'm in therapy to cope with some of my discomfort, and I feel I've done a lot. Every once in a while I need to ask him for reassurance.

I like that our sex life has improved, his mood and substance use has improved, and our communication has improved. You need to be honest, patient, and understanding that strong feelings will arise.

—Sarah, 31

WHERE DO WE GO FROM HERE?

The last few pages may have been hard to read. It might have felt as if this chapter was nothing more than a laundry list of every worry you're holding right now. I get that. The decision to move through discomfort is a powerful act. Alternately, perhaps you're feeling relieved to have your feelings and experiences validated. Either way, you're not alone, and I am so grateful that you've kept turning the pages and made it here. I can't promise that the rest of what we will do together will resolve your worries. You are the ultimate authority on your life and experiences, and only you can ultimately decide what is right and best for you. What I can do is give you context, information, options, opportunities, and hope.

We are going to look at the realities that underlie the fears explored here: what it means (and doesn't mean) to be kinky; more about how BDSM and kink can be expressed by people who are attracted to these activities; worries about inadequacy or embarrassment; and differences in desire and concerns about being "too boring" or "not enough." And finally, we're going to take a serious look at what it means if you come to the end of this learning process and realize that this just isn't where you want to be anymore. But for now? I'd like to offer four guiding principles for how you and your partner might try to communicate about these topics while you undertake this journey:

1. Recognize that both of you may be feeling the same emotions (anger, confusion, betrayal, guilt/shame, fear) but for different reasons and at different times.

2. Respond to actual behaviors (if any) rather than fantasies or desires.

3. Understand that new information about your partner expands what you know about them but does not change who they actually are. (Note: As you work through some of the exercises contained within, you may notice this applies to *you* as well.)

4. You set your own pace and your own boundaries as we move forward through this book. Go as fast or as slow as you need and take time to process as you talk and learn.

THE EMPATHY INTERVIEW

When you feel ready, set aside some time to ask your partner the questions below and to answer their questions as well. The purpose of these questions is not to elicit factual information about the specific behaviors or kinks but rather to gain insights into your respective emotional states before and after the disclosure/discovery. My recommendation is that you do the Empathy Interview exercise at least three times on different days and at different times, because your answers will evolve and expand as you put time between yourselves and the moment of discovery/disclosure. These changes don't typically represent deception but rather the clarity that comes with distance and de-escalation of conflict in the immediate aftermath of the discovery/disclosure.

Questions to Ask the Secret Holder

1. How did it feel, physically and emotionally, to have to hide this aspect of yourself?

2. What did you fear most about me knowing this about you?

3. How did you hope I would react to this information?

4. When did you first know that this was something that you needed/were curious about?

5. Who else knows about this part of you?

6. Why did you keep this a secret?

7. Where do you want us to go from here?

Questions to Ask the Secret Discoverer

1. How did it feel, physically and emotionally, to learn about this part of me?

2. Have you ever kept a secret from someone else? Can you tell me more about why you held the secret?

3. Have you ever experienced deep fear, embarrassment, or shame?

4. What, if anything, has this information changed about me in your eyes?

5. What is your biggest fear in this moment?

6. What do you wish you knew more about?

7. Where do you want us to go from here?

In the introduction we talked a bit about what's "normal" versus what's "normative." That idea will be expanded in the chapters that follow. The important thing is that we begin to create a picture of what healthy kink expression can (not should, not must!) look like and to offer a framework to understand that most BDSM fantasies and desires are normal, healthy, and safe. One of the most important elements of my clinical work with clients is the process of helping them understand that fact. Once we've worked through those fears—the concerns about being dirty, sinful, broken, or wrong—once we understand what everyday kink might look like, from there we can begin the process of finding those places where our vanilla desires overlap with aspects of BDSM. We begin with empathy. From there, we educate, explore, and (perhaps) expand.

MORE TO READ ON THIS TOPIC

Boundaries: Where You End and I Begin

Anne Katherine

Erotic Integrity: How to Be True to Yourself Sexually

Claudia Six

Sinless Sex: A Challenge to Religions

William R. Strayton

2

Meet Your Kinkster!

As we discussed in the introduction, BDSM (the Swiss Army knife of acronyms!) encompasses three unique forms of consensual power exchange: bondage and discipline, the exchange of *control*; dominance and submission, the exchange of *authority*; and sadism and masochism, the exchange of *sensation*. In this chapter we're going to learn more about the psychology of kink and what we know about the nature of kinky people as individuals and kinky relationships. Many forms of BDSM can be enjoyed by an individual without the involvement of a partner. For example, rope aficionados (called riggers) who enjoy self-bondage can create elaborate rope harnesses to wear under their clothing or even perform amazing feats of self-suspension, which can be quite impressive to see. Likewise, there are many kink-identified folks who create a discipline practice—a structured way of moving through their day—and hold themselves accountable for any slipups in this orderly routine without the input of others. Along the same line, there are solo masochists who incorporate intense sensations into their masturbation and don't rely on a partner to provide the experiences they enjoy.

Things become a bit more complicated when we consider dominance and submission (often abbreviated D/s). Because this centers around the consensual giving and receiving of control from one person to another, it can be difficult to create the desired authority dynamic in isolation. D/s is relational by its nature, and people on both sides of the slash—both dominant and submissive personalities—may feel adrift or unfulfilled if they don't have a partner who balances them out and allows them to have that back-and-forth power exchange that they find so satisfying.

BDSM BASICS

As someone who makes my living through words—in the counseling room, in the media, or on the page—I know how important it is to make sure that the words I use are understood by the folks I'm talking to. For example, if I ask a client to picture the sky, I might assume that they're visualizing a pale blue, sunny expanse dotted with clouds, whereas they might be imagining a vivid sunset full of just about every color *but* blue. We're both thinking of the sky, but what we mean by "sky" is different—and that's when misunderstandings, miscommunication, and conflict can arise.

Just like the sky, the term *kink* encompasses many subjects and many variations on each subject. That's why it's important before we talk more about kinky people and what science and psychology can tell us about them, to make sure that we're on the same page with what it is, exactly, that we're talking about. In social science, we call these "operant definitions"—the definitions we agree to use up front, to make sure that everyone is talking about the same thing when they discuss a topic or issue. So, let's start with a vocabulary lesson. Not because you don't know what some of these terms are already but so we understand what we mean and how we're using them in this particular conversation together.

Let's start with the word I've thrown around most already, *kink*, and its descriptive version, *kinky*. What exactly do I mean when I call something (or someone) kinky? At the most basic level, **kink is simply anything that falls outside of the social and cultural idea of "normal" sexual expression and relationship style.** What we consider kinky varies depending upon where you live and how you were raised, and it changes over time. Things that we consider erotic today, such as stockings and garters, were just . . . undergarments . . . not so long ago. Likewise, the rather mundane (to us) idea of a husband performing oral sex on his wife? It was a scandalous act that could be prosecuted in court until fairly recently![1] In other words, what is kinky is often whatever is most novel within a given social group at any given time. Today, when most people describe something as kinky, they're thinking of two things: fetishes and BDSM.

There are some terms specific to kink that you may encounter throughout our conversations—both within these pages and with each other. Just like the sky, these are common words that have unique meanings within the BDSM community. Knowing what these words mean in the context of kink and being able to use them as you negotiate your own learning, boundary-setting, and explorations will help to minimize confusion and increase understanding between you and your partner. What follows is a quick primer of kinky key terms:

Fetish: A strong sexual interest in or desire for an object or body part that is not typically seen as sexual. **All fetishes fall under the umbrella of kink, but not all fetishists practice BDSM.**

Top: The person who takes control/authority over their partner or who provides their partner with intense sensation for a negotiated time period ranging from a few moments to a lifetime. The topping partner may be referred to with an honorific that may be gendered and that reflects the relationship dynamic. Examples: Dominant/Domina/Domme, Master, Trainer, Caregiver, Owner, Sir, Madam, Mistress, Leader, and so forth.

Bottom: The person who gives up control/authority to their partner or who receives intense sensation from them for a negotiated time period ranging from a few moments to a lifetime. The bottoming partner may be referred to with a diminutive that may be gendered and that reflects the relationship dynamic. Examples: submissive, slave, pet, little, boy/girl, follower, and so forth.

Dynamic: The specific power-exchange agreement that has been negotiated between partners. Someone might have a D/s dynamic, for example, or a caregiver/little dynamic. The details of a BDSM relationship dynamic will vary and may evolve or be renegotiated over time.

Munch/Slosh: A public event where people who identify as kinky can gather to converse, make friends, and socialize. These typically occur in restaurants (munch) or bars (slosh) and do not involve any physical contact or BDSM play.

Play: Another term for BDSM activities. These may be individual, partnered, or group and may or may not involve sexual or physical contact between the people involved.

Scene: A negotiated BDSM encounter between two or more individuals. A scene usually occurs in person and may or may not include sexual intercourse (or even physical contact) between the people involved.

Play Partner: A "friend with benefits"—someone with whom another may engage in BDSM play or sexual activities but where no romantic or committed relationship is expected.

Play Party: A public or private event, organized by members of the BDSM community, where kinksters can socialize and watch or engage in public BDSM scenes using tools and equipment that they likely don't have at home. Many of these occur at BDSM conferences and conventions or private membership clubs.

Ethical Nonmonogamy: An umbrella term that encompasses both polyamory—the practice of having romantic/emotional/ sexual relationships with more than one partner at a time—and swinging—the practice of having sexual relationships or encounters outside of a committed relationship with the full knowledge and consent of all involved.

Leather Family: A "chosen family" bound by shared LGBTQIA+ history as well as protocols and rituals unique to the family. Familial bonds may be nonsexual but very close-knit, are typically grounded in a master/slave hierarchy, and are by invitation only.

Queer Platonic Relationship: A committed relationship that may include shared finances, shared household, or coparenting but is nonsexual and potentially nonromantic.

ARE KINKY PEOPLE BROKEN?

As we discussed at the start of this chapter, what is considered kinky relies a great deal on the time and culture in which the behavior occurs. Many practices that would be seen as extreme even among members of the BDSM community today—for example, whipping oneself bloody, wearing clothing designed to irritate the skin for days, or engaging in grotesque acts of degradation—were considered routine elements of life in a medieval monastery.[2] And yet one of the earliest mentions of kinky people occurs in the writings of a German inquisitor who wrote that those who derived pleasure from the deviant act of self-flagellation were burned at the stake.[3] When historical observers sought to understand behavior that we might today call kinky, they often relied on the motivations of the actors—on one hand, masochistic acts for sexual pleasure could lead to prison or the stake; on the other, extreme acts of mortification and humiliation intended to purify the spirit might destine the person for sainthood.

Brief History of Kinky Sexology

The Enlightenment and the rise of the scientific era shifted the Western/ European conversation about sex and sexuality away from a faith-based "saints and sinners" perspective and toward the notion that our understanding of healthy sexuality should be informed by our understanding of medicine and the philosophy of natural law. Unfortunately the common understanding of what was "natural" was heavily informed by the opinions of white European men. Notions of what was medically and socially acceptable were influenced by beliefs in strict class hierarchy (it's near impossible to engage in consensual power exchange when one person is *genuinely* lacking in autonomy and power) and the inferior status of women, who were seen as naturally weaker, less intelligent, and less sexual than their male counterparts.

And because this was the "modern" age? The appropriate way to address those who deviated from what was understood to be the natural order was through medical intervention. The German neuropsychiatrist Richard von Krafft-Ebing encouraged modern experts to try to differentiate between perverse acts and perverse instincts, to try to "avoid the danger of covering simple immorality with the cloak of disease."[4] Doctors prescribed any number of devices meant to discourage masturbation, often by inflicting pain to the aroused genitals as a deterrent to the dreaded disease "spermatorrhoea." This was basically the masculine version of hysteria, a belief that much of women's bad, confusing, or inappropriate behavior was caused by the uterus wandering around their body and causing all kinds of mental and medical distress. Needless to say, hysteria is a ridiculous and thoroughly debunked idea; and at the time, it was basically an attempt by the early twentieth-century psychoanalyst Sigmund Freud to use medical jargon and the power of "modern science" to enforce what people of the day considered to be socially appropriate femininity.[5] In fact, the medical concern about female sexuality was so great that women who enjoyed sex to a degree that the men in their lives deemed to be unfeminine might have their abnormal desire treated with a clitoridectomy—the surgical removal of their clitoris.[6] And people of all genders who engaged in "unnatural" relationships (which at this time meant anything that challenged strict notions of social hierarchy, modesty, and heterosexuality) could find themselves hospitalized in an asylum where they would receive the very latest in medical treatments, ranging from vocational training and social etiquette courses to ice baths, electric shocks, and even lobotomies.[7]

From the moral framework of the Middle Ages to the natural law of the eighteenth and nineteenth centuries, the twentieth century introduced the idea that perhaps we could understand why people did the things they did (good, bad, and confusing) through the new tools of behavioral health and psychology. Instead of starting from their own ideas of what appropriate behavior *should* look like, doctors and social scientists began to conduct research to figure out what "normal" actually was. The definition of homosexuality evolved from "an abnormal or perverted appetite toward the opposite sex" to our more mundane understanding of the term today.[8] The German physician and sexologist Magnus Hirschfeld's research into the nature of homosexuality (which would later be burned by the Nazis) introduced the idea that same-sex desire was a natural state for many. The American biologist Alfred Kinsey's famous reports blew readers' minds when he revealed that many of their friends and neighbors admitted not only to masturbating (gasp!) but to trying and enjoying various forms of BDSM play. The pioneering sex researchers William Masters and Virginia Johnson studied the female orgasm and proved that cis women's bodies were just as sexually responsive as cis men.

As this groundbreaking research gave us a new understanding of what constitutes *normal* and *natural* (two very subjective terms) behavior, so too our understanding of what should be considered problematic behavior has evolved: first, simply by shifting our language to recognize that problematic behavior isn't necessarily unnatural or abnormal; and second, by focusing more on how this problematic behavior impacts the lives of the person engaging in the behavior and the people around them. Today, the DSM-5 instructs clinicians that BDSM activities should only be considered a problem if it:

- causes the person significant distress (which usually takes the form of intense guilt or shame about their desires);

- causes significant distress to others around them, such as by violating their consent or causing other harm; or,

- interferes with important areas of their life, such as work or parenting.[9]

In other words? We no longer call a behavior harmful simply because some find it sinful, unnatural, or weird. It only rises to the level of a problem when the behavior itself is causing *actual* problems. Otherwise? We just call it kinky.

What We Know about Kink and Mental Health

Okay, now that we understand that what is considered "normal" or "problematic" changes over time and varies by culture and social group, what does that tell us about kinky people *today*? Are *they* normal? Crazy? Criminal? It's all well and good that Kinsey, Hirschfeld, and the gang were asking those questions back in the 1930s into the 1950s, but what does present-day research tell us about BDSM and mental health? One report that analyzed data from a national survey for the *Journal of Sexual Medicine* said,

> *There is no evidence that BDSM practitioners in general suffer from any particular form of psychological disturbance and in fact they seem to be mentally and emotionally well-adjusted.*[10]

In 2016, the Alternative Sexualities Health Research Alliance (TASHRA) conducted a sweeping survey of BDSM practitioners that focused specifically on learning more about the health (both physical and mental) of kinky folks. When they reviewed over thirty years of research into BDSM and its practitioners, the research team found no difference in the rates of anxiety, obsessive-compulsive disorder, authoritarianism, or other forms of general psychological distress between kinky people and their vanilla peers. TASHRA did note a difference in the depression rates between kinky and nonkinky people: **41.8 percent of kinky people reported receiving a diagnosis of depression at some point in their lives, versus 16.6 percent of the general population.**[11]

This difference could be explained by the theory of minority stress, which is experienced by many sexual minorities. Minority stress is the psychological distress felt when someone experiences prejudice, rejection, discrimination, or victimization because of an aspect of their identity that is different from the dominant culture. It's exacerbated by the mental and emotional energy it takes to conceal or hide the part of themselves that they feel has been rejected and the internalized messages of shame that they might learn from these experiences.[12]

TASHRA also noticed the rate of post-traumatic stress disorder (PTSD) within the BDSM community: **17.98 percent of kinky people reported a diagnosis of PTSD at some point in their lives, versus 6.8 percent of the general population.** What's fascinating about this is the fact that **kinky people do not report higher rates of trauma than their vanilla peers.** One explanation for this might be that the expectations for a kinky scene—such as ongoing, affirmative consent; bodily autonomy; negotiation; and boundary setting—might appeal to some trauma survivors who find BDSM to be a form of self-care or healing. After all, **85.16 percent of kinky people told TASHRA that BDSM had a positive influence on their lives.**[13]

Additionally, clinician and kink researcher Elyssa Helfer theorizes that the same self-awareness and communications skills necessary to successfully negotiate a power-exchange scene are themselves a part of what enables research study participants to acknowledge their emotional struggles:

There is no evidence that these results (higher levels of depression and PTSD) are the result of participation in BDSM—the whole correlation doesn't equal causation thing. Kinky people are often incredibly communicative, open, and exploratory. These are people who are naturally in touch with themselves and their feelings because in order to participate in kink in a healthy way, they have to have pretty significant insight into who they are and how they express themselves. To be a kinky person, and the kind of person open and honest enough to participate in research, could mean that we are dealing with people who are more in touch with who they are and who have done more personal exploration than the general population.[14]

WHAT KIND OF PEOPLE ENJOY BDSM?

As mentioned in the introduction, kinky people tend to be well educated, work in professional or white-collar jobs, and generally identify as religiously secular.[15] While most report being in monogamous relationships, they are more inclined toward ethical nonmonogamy than their vanilla peers and might interpret "monogamy" a bit more creatively (see chapter 7). Most surveys have found that the BDSM community is predominantly Caucasian, but this is likely due more to sample biases and challenges in conducting this kind of research rather than being a true picture of the kinky world.

Ali Hébert and Angela Weaver researched what kinds of personalities enjoy BDSM. Their findings confirmed the statement about positive mental health published in the *Journal of Sexual Medicine*: the kinky people they studied (who they divided up into general categories of dominant and submissive) **"fell within the normal range for Honesty-Humility, Emotionality, Extraversion, Agreeableness, and Conscientiousness. . . . Desire for Control, Self-Esteem, Life Satisfaction and Empathy."**[16] In other words, BDSM is not something enjoyed by some strange subset of people who can be identified by a unique constellation of personality traits that spell "kinky."

While we can't look at a group of people and sort them into kinky and nonkinky clusters based on their personalities, Hébert and Weaver were able to identify some differences between more dominant and more submissive personalities. You may not be surprised to learn that **dominant types tend to be more extroverted than their submissive peers, while submissive types tend to rate a bit higher in emotionality.** This seems to fit the archetypical picture of D/s, with the strong, assertive, perhaps even demanding Dom and their quieter, more affectionate sub. Perhaps also not surprisingly, **submissive personality types scored higher than their dominant counterparts in openness to new ideas**, which makes perfect sense for a group of people who enjoy relinquishing control (temporarily or otherwise) to the creative machinations of a partner. A good thing, too, since **dominants score higher than submissives in desire for control.**

So what's the takeaway here—*kinky people look just like everyone else*? Isn't that what Wednesday Addams said about homicidal maniacs? Yes! And that's what makes this such an important point, because when we see

BDSM and kink portrayed in the media, it so often takes the form of something "othered" and strange. Kinky people are not intrinsically damaged or dangerous people. They are no more likely to be diagnosed with psychological sadism or masochism, problematic attachment styles, or antisocial tendencies than their vanilla peers.[17] The reality is that **BDSM is enjoyed by psychologically healthy people with healthy personalities**, who simply enjoy the novelty, sensations, and intimacy that kinky play affords them.

WHY DO PEOPLE LIKE THIS STUFF?

Okay, but why? Why do psychologically healthy people choose to spend their time giving and receiving painful stimulation, letting others make personal decisions for them, tying their partners up in ropes and chains? What is the appeal of having sex in a kiddie pool full of butterscotch pudding or wearing a head-to-toe latex bodysuit? For many nonkinky people, the perceived oddness of kinky play is a mental block that seems insurmountable. They can't possibly imagine what an adult man finds enjoyable about dressing up like a pony and pulling a cart around a track. Like Elvis's peanut butter, bacon, and banana sandwiches—the combination just seems weird to some folks. Needless to say, this is a question that social scientists and sexologists have been exploring for many years now, and they've discovered a variety of benefits that BDSM affords to those who enjoy partaking. Here is a partial list of just some of the benefits that researchers have identified:

Physical Benefits of Kink

- endorphin rush/natural high[18]

- increased serotonin levels[19]

- chronic pain management[20]

- heightened sensory experiences[21]

- increased body awareness[22]

- reduced physical stress (cortisol levels)[23]

- reduced inflammation[24]

- experience of being in a "flow state"[25]

- increased sexual satisfaction (when their partner knew about their desires)[26]

Psycho-Emotional Benefits of Kink

- autonomy and a sense of control[27]

- personal growth[28]

- enhanced sense of resilience[29]

- community connections[30]

- psychological release[31]

- a break from everyday roles[32]

- freedom to be yourself[33]

- a sense of power (dominant/top)[34]

- opportunities to relinquish control (submissive/bottom)[35]

- improved self-esteem/body confidence[36]

- ability to role-play and explore other identities[37]

- reduced sense of shame[38]

- healthy outlet for potentially unhealthy desires[39]

- a tool for processing trauma[40]

- respect for and inclusion of diverse gender roles[41]

Relational Benefits of Kink

- adding fun and variety to the relationship[42]

- improved romantic relationships[43]

- pleasure from pleasuring others[44]

- increased sense of relationship closeness[45]

- improved communication between partners[46]

- deepened trust[47]

- stronger relationship attachment/security[48]

Mixed Desire

I've always been into bondage and domination but not sadomasochism. I learned about BDSM really young, honestly—probably around eleven or twelve. My dad had all the classic books—stuff like *The Story of O*—hidden on his bookshelf, and I stole them. Also, I was on the internet unsupervised, with the writing skills of someone much older, so I practically lived in AOL chat rooms. I like being taken care of, cared for—a gentle dominance with me as the follower. I don't like pain. Don't spank me. Nothing like that. I do like bondage and the feeling of being restricted. Metal, leather, rope—it's all good! In a perfect world, my partner and I would have a casual D/s dynamic—reminding me to take my vitamins or drink enough water . . . and then also pushing my boundaries a bit—letting me have that adrenaline rush of doing something that might be a little scary.

For most of my dating life, I was meeting people on BDSM-focused sites like FetLife, so they already knew. I met my now-husband and fell in love, even though he didn't come out of that world. When we first got together, we talked about it a little bit, but it was mostly me feeling him out gently. It's hard sometimes to introduce the idea of kink because you never know what someone is going to say or if you'll be on the same page. He's so respectful of boundaries that it's insane. I told him not to pinch my butt once over a decade ago and he's never done it since.

Now that said, I've also asked for us to schedule playdates—times when we can do some of the things, like rope, that I enjoy so much. It hasn't worked out well. It's just not a priority for him, which makes it easy to forget. And then I feel ashamed sometimes, because I want all these things that are weird and a bit dirty and he's just blasé and perfectly content with normal, vanilla sex for the rest of his life. He's doing it for me. And me leading has always made me feel ashamed to be asking for things. It can be frustrating. He wants to do forty minutes of gentle foreplay—kissing, fondling, touching—and at minute five I am *so bored*. I want rougher sex, bondage, him telling me what to do . . . ANYTHING!

The bright side of our relationship is that he is extremely affectionate—sometimes more than I can handle. I can always have a hug if I want one. I feel safe with him. He will support my weird ideas and go along with anything I want to do for myself without question. I definitely married up! He's an amazing person, super supportive, and genuinely concerned for my well-being and happiness. On the other side? The harder part? I'm not sure when I'm pushing past his comfort zone. He's so willing to say yes that he doesn't say no often enough. His limits would be *very much* clearer in a D/s relationship. I wish he knew that I appreciate being told no because then I know where the boundaries are . . . and that the best way to start something frisky with me is to grab a pair of handcuffs! I wouldn't want to try anything new because I'd worry that I'd be pushing limits he won't acknowledge.

You know that saying "you can lead a horse to water but you can't make it drink"? FUCKING DRINK, DAMN IT! I have sent so many ideas, offered compromises, sent stories, really exposed myself and it just . . . disappears into the ether. It's so frustrating. Meet me halfway. Be clearer about the things you'd want to do or be willing to try. Come up with some ideas of your own—that's a big one, honestly. I feel like it's been me putting ideas out all the time and that leaves me feeling exposed and then it's not reciprocated. Listen to your person's requests (and not just once) and do some reading and research of your own. That can be fun too—see if anything appeals.

—Melanie, 39

IS KINK ABUSE?

The shortest answer to this question is simply no. BDSM is the consensual, negotiated exchange of power by people who enjoy giving and receiving power. If the situation does not include those key components: consent, negotiation, and enjoyment? Then we're no longer talking about kink. We're probably describing abuse. What do those elements look like in a healthy kink dynamic?

Consent is perhaps the core value of the BDSM community. So much so that the National Leather Alliance founded the BDSM community's first anti–domestic violence program way back in 1975, to address concerns about consent in kink spaces.[49] When kinksters talk about consent, they don't just mean permission from one's partner to have sex with them. Consent in this context includes informed consent about one's partner's health status, whether or not they have other sex or play partners, and permission to engage in various forms of BDSM play either together or with others, among other topics. Transparency is the expected ethical default within most kink communities, and secret-keeping is often seen as a form of consent violation.

That's where negotiation comes into play. It is common for kinky people who are interested in dating each other, or even having a one-time scene at an event, to engage in some fairly direct boundary negotiation up front. For many more vanilla folks who haven't experienced this process firsthand, the uniquely specific nature of negotiation can feel very forward, even presumptuous. Asking someone about their preferred power dynamic, whether or not they enjoy various sexual or sensory activities, and what names they enjoy being called can seem off-putting. In the world of BDSM, this is a fairly typical part of the courtship process, similar to making sure an intriguing individual on OkCupid shares your taste in entertainment and hobbies before asking them out on a date.

Negotiation carries over into long-term relationships as well. Some kinky couples will create a written contract, codifying their dynamic and laying out the rules, practices, words, and limits they have mutually agreed to follow. Other partnerships are less formal but create space for regular check-in conversations to discuss what's working, what could be better, and what changes they might want to make to the dynamic. People grow, evolve, and change with time, and our desires and limits shift with us. Negotiation in BDSM is a fluid process. Agreements are revisited again and again to make sure that the present relationship reflects who and where they are right now and not where they were five years ago or where they hope to be in six months.

The negotiations process is what ensures that kinky play is enjoyable for everyone involved. It allows the participants to describe what they enjoy—without judgment or shame—and to create scenes that fulfill these desires for them. I'm saying "enjoyment" here and not "pleasure" because different people experience kink in different ways. Some of the BDSM activities that people enjoy are not physically pleasurable and may even be degrading, dirty, or painful. And that's okay! A common catchphrase in the BDSM community is "Your kink's not my kink, but your kink's okay." We don't need to understand why someone enjoys what they enjoy, and we are not obligated to participate in it with them. We simply need to respect the fact that it is enjoyable for them and ensure that our partners have enjoyable experiences when they are with us, whatever form that takes.

Red Flags and Warning Signs

When people are forced—either by pressure, force, or surprise—into activities that they do not find enjoyable, that is a consent violation and a red flag for abuse. Unfortunately there are people within and outside the kink community who use the language of BDSM to justify abusive behavior or to gaslight their partners into staying in unhealthy dynamics. When you have a population of people who truly enjoy playing with authority and control in their relationships, who savor intense sensations that others might find painful or scary, there will be predators who seek to exploit these desires.

Being able to differentiate between consensual kink and intimate-partner abuse starts with a mindful awareness of consent, negotiation, and enjoyment. The absence of any one of these three might be a warning light to those involved; the absence of more than one indicates a serious problem. It can be difficult to point to a mainstream resource such as the Duluth model's Power and Control Wheel—a tool to help explain the different ways an abusive partner can use power and control to manipulate a relationship—because they highlight some behaviors that might be quite fun within a negotiated, consensual, power-exchange relationship. That said, there are some actions that are abusive no matter what kind of relationship you have and some behaviors that are best described as abusive BDSM. A non-exhaustive list follows, but keep in mind: if it's not consensual, negotiated, and enjoyed by everyone involved? It's not kink; it's abuse.

Abusive in Any Dynamic

- prevents communication with friends or family
- listens in on phone calls/screens texts/emails
- withholds financial support
- denies that problematic behavior occurred
- threatens self-harm or suicide if relationship ends/changes
- destroys property
- threatens to harm children or pets
- body/disability shaming

Abuse Masquerading as BDSM

- denial of basic needs (food, water, rest)
- deliberately unsafe play
- deliberately violating negotiated limits
- ignoring safe words
- inappropriate boundaries/scene confusion
- punishment or scene play when the Top is angry
- using power-exchange punishment to address nonkink-related conflicts
- failure to stop scene/seek treatment for injury
- body/disability shaming (outside of negotiated boundaries)
- threatening to "out" partner if they don't comply

I hope that this chapter has offered some context for what "normal," healthy, consensual kink can look like. BDSM and kink are vast and contain such a wide variety of relationship styles, ways of connecting, sensory experiences, and sexy play that it would be impossible to offer a complete picture of all of kink here . . . or anywhere. That's why there is so much great content created about these communities! One book can never (and should never) be enough. That said, one key thing to take away from this chapter is the difference between kink in any form and abuse. If you recognize yourself, your partner, or your relationship in the list above, please take that awareness very seriously. If you don't, I'd like you to consider the idea that kink is not only safe and pleasurable but it can be a force for good in our lives and relationships. Sometimes knowing that—even believing that—is not enough, however. Sometimes we worry that even if kink is perfectly fine and totally acceptable, our partner's kinks might present a problem for our relationships specifically. Let's talk about what it might mean to understand that kink is healthy and safe . . . and to still feel like it's not a fit for us.

MORE TO READ ON THIS TOPIC

A Lover's Pinch: A Cultural History of Sadomasochism

Peter Tupper

Screw the Roses, Send Me the Thorns: The Romance and Sexual Sorcery of Sadomasochism

Philip Miller and Molly Devon

SM 101: A Realistic Introduction

Jay Wiseman

3

Feeling Vanilla in a Thirty-One-Flavors Kind of World

BDSM and kink have become pervasive themes within pop culture. Madonna and Rhianna, Alexander McQueen and E. L. James's *Fifty Shades of Grey* all have raised our general cultural comfort level with the images and icons of BDSM. Because of this, there are many people who are able to receive their partners' disclosures with openhearted acceptance and fearless affirmation. Ironically, where a vanilla person might experience conflict is in the way this new knowledge can challenge how they feel about *themselves*. For better or worse, many of us carry a self-concept that is at least partially defined by our relationships with others: We look to our coworkers as a measure of our own professional skill. We tend to see our children's behavior as representative of our parenting skills. And we use the quality of our relationship in any given moment to determine whether or not we are being a "good" partner. When we learn something about our partner that challenges our understanding of them? We might react not by pushing them away but rather by asking, "Wait . . . what's wrong with *me*?"

WHY DIDN'T I SEE IT?

In my practice, I see a great number of couples who have decided to seek out counseling after some form of secret-keeping causes a fissure in the relationship. These secrets are not always sexual in nature. I've worked with couples reeling from the fallout of substance-use challenges, gambling problems, problematic friendships, even medical diagnoses. The consistent question I hear from the person who has discovered this boundary violation is "Why didn't I see it?" We like to think that we know our partners so well that if they had something significant happening in their lives, we'd just *know*. And when we find out that there was something going on that we did not see, it can be hard not to think of that blind spot as a failing in ourselves.

Michael Slepian, one of the few researchers studying the psychology of secrecy, defines secret-keeping as "not just as the moment of actively withholding information, but also having the intention to keep something secret from another person—even when that other person isn't physically present."[1] His team identified thirty-eight common secret types ranging from affairs to surprise parties and discovered that "about 92% of people have a secret in at least one of those categories, and the average person is currently keeping secrets in 13 of those categories."[2]

Most of us move through the world assuming that the people we interact with are generally honest people. We expect a certain degree of transparency, and we tend to look at withholding information as a form of deception. And yet Slepian's research flips that assumption on its head! After all, if nearly everyone we encounter is keeping a dozen possible secrets, how can we possibly assume either ill intentions from them or lack of insight for ourselves? The reality is simply this: nearly everyone keeps some information about themselves and their lives private. Most of these secrets are benign. And the notion that we could somehow tell when someone is holding a single specific secret from us feels like an awfully unfair expectation to have for ourselves.

Where we do pick up on cues that our partner might be keeping something from us, it's often not because we're finding "evidence" of deception: unexplained receipts or missing money, mysterious phone calls and lipstick on collars. More often, our attunement to our partner allows us to pick up on the subtle physiological ways that secret-keeping impacts a person. We might notice disruptions in their sleep, complaints about upset stomachs or other gastrointestinal distress, the distractibility that can come when someone is ruminating on their thoughts.[3] If we notice these things and ask our partner about them, we are offered reassurance that everything is fine. And I believe that these reassurances are genuine! Most folks don't make a connection between their personal/relational behaviors and physical discomfort. In the absence of this self-insight (or genuine medical concerns), they are sincere in their reassurances. Unfortunately, when the secret comes out, these passing conversations can feel like gaslighting in hindsight.

The pain that comes when a secret is revealed lies in the ways we retroactively evaluate these interactions and ascribe new meaning to them. Often we come to believe that the act of holding the secret was a statement on our value as a partner. After all, if they really loved us, they wouldn't have held something back at all, right? Counterintuitively, research has found that people are more likely to keep secrets from people they care most about, as a way of protecting and preserving the relationship. Overall, keeping the secret was seen as creating a slight amount of distance between the secret-keeper and the target person. But among participants in high-quality relationships, keeping the secret was seen as having a positive impact on the level of closeness.[4] The researchers described this as the protective function of secrecy.

Likewise, sharing a secret can strengthen relationships. The act of opening up to another person and telling them something we had previously held private has been shown to increase feelings of intimacy and connection experienced by the secret hearer. When a secret shared is received with compassion and support and without judgment, the one making the disclosure also feels closer to the person they've told. And perhaps unsurprisingly, the more extraordinary the secret, the closer and more connected the parties feel once it's been voiced.[5] This is the outcome that many couples experience when an interest in BDSM or kink is revealed. When the vanilla listener responds with curiosity and calm, the kinky sharer is able to reveal this part of their world to them, building an open line of communication, companionship, and connection that did not exist before their desires were disclosed—an ideal outcome for any relationship flavor.

DOES THIS MEAN THEY DON'T WANT ME?

Regardless of whether we are kinky or vanilla, it can be difficult to hear the details of our partner's desires. The idea that they have fantasies that involve scenarios we might not envision for ourselves or even fantasies that don't involve us at all can leave us feeling excluded from our partner's desires. From there, it can feel like a natural leap to assume that our partner doesn't desire us at all. We want to know that our partner wants us, craves us. We want to know we have a place even in their wildest fantasies. It can feel like a violation to learn that our partner fantasizes about other people, particularly when their fantasy is less romantic than sexual—especially when they disclose fantasies that we find ourselves unwilling or incapable of sharing with them.[6] These disclosures can leave us thinking, "If that's what they want . . . do they even want *me* at all?"

Fantasy

Sex therapist Barry McCarthy, the author of over a dozen books on desire and sexuality, said, "Erotic fantasies are, by definition, not socially acceptable. It is the rare person who fantasizes about having mission position sex, in their bed, with their partner. Erotic fantasy is where we explore the scenarios we cannot speak out loud."[7] Many of us revel in the private power to explore scenarios or ideas that perhaps we'd never want to pursue in real life but that feel super sexy as a hypothetical. We can indulge in fantasies that may be off-putting or even impossible in real life. The sticking point for some kinky-vanilla mixed-desire relationships is when the world of BDSM opens up the possibility of acting out fantasies that might otherwise stay within the realm of the imagination. When we don't see ourselves and our desires represented in our partner's fantasies, we may wonder if we are at risk of being replaced by someone (or something) who is. These feelings of insecurity and anxiety can be compounded with confusion when we introduce kink into the mix and recognize that sometimes people fantasize about things that seem, well, downright fantastical to us. In my practice, I have worked with many folks who have expressed concern about their partners' fantasies about . . .

OTHER PEOPLE: No one likes to think that our partner lusts after others. Discovering that they enjoy erotic material that may feature folks who look and act nothing like us can be a blow to our self-esteem. Particularly when the differences are so stark (race, body type, gender) that we feel we can't possibly compete. It can be hard not to assume that if the other person represents whatever our partner finds sexy or attractive, and we don't look like that person, then our partner doesn't find us sexy or attractive. Yet these differences often represent a quest for variety and a thirst for novelty rather than a hard-and-fast statement about what kinds of people or bodies we find appealing, particularly since most people will find multiple bodies attractive over the course of their lives: "When asked how many sexual partners would be ideal in the next 30 years, men report an ideal of 2–9 partners while women report an ideal preference for 1–4 partners."[8] The Centers for Disease Control and Prevention (CDC) reports that among people aged twenty-five to forty-four, men report an average of six sexual partners, while women have four.[9] It's no wonder, then, that most of us fantasize at one point or another about having sex with someone (or several someones) other than our partner—or even about having sex with our partner and other people! After all, group-sex scenarios such as threesomes, gang bangs, or orgies are the most common sexual fantasy for people of both genders, according to psychologist Justin Lehmiller, the author of *Tell Me What You Want*.[10]

ROUGH SEX: Speaking of gang bangs! Coming in at number two on Lehmiller's list of most popular sexual fantasies is BDSM and rough sex. We've already been talking quite a bit about the relational nature of BDSM and how kink can be used as a positive force in the lives of those who enjoy it. These are useful things to know! But they can feel rather academic when we come face to face with fantasy material that depicts scenes of aggressive behavior such as slapping and hair pulling and rough, far-from-romantic sex. It can feel scary to think about someone getting off on violence. We wonder what it is about them—some hidden darkness we never saw before—that makes this kind of thing appealing. We wonder if they want to hurt us or be hurt by us; and if so, we worry about what these violent tendencies say about the way they view us.

The answers to these questions tend to be yes and no. *Yes*—people who enjoy rough sex like engaging in rough sex with other people who like rough sex. In other words? It's hot to rough up someone who enjoys the experience. *No*—our partner's daydreams about aggressive sex are not a comment on the love or respect they have for us. Roy F. Baumeister used the phrase "hurt, not harm" when writing about the goal of sadomasochism.[11] The pleasure lies in the fact that the person on the receiving end of the scene—whether it's a trail of tiny, tickling kisses down their belly or a dozen lashes with a single-tail whip—is *enjoying* the sensations they are experiencing. They like the hurt. But no one is trying to actively cause them harm. Baumeister's research shows that when actual harm is inflicted by the topping partner in a scene, that pulls both partners out of the moment and tends to shift them into a "soothe and heal" direction.

The goal of enjoyable hurt has been thwarted, and they move to respond to the harm that has been caused—because they in fact do value their partner and want them to have a safe and pleasurable experience of rough sexual use. For many kinksters, fantasies about rough sex are just that—fantasy. It's hot to think about or watch in private, but they might not ever want to act out these scenes with someone they care about. And rarely are rough-sex fantasies commentary on the love, affection, and value they hold for their partner.

OBJECTS: In some ways, sexual desire for objects is the most clichéd form of BDSM expression. In my experience, whenever the topic of kink arises, the question "What, like a foot fetish?" isn't far behind. This might be because feet are indeed the most popular fetish object. Or it might be because culturally we use objects such as high heels, corsets, leather, and latex as a visual cue for eroticism and so naturally come to associate these same objects with sex and sexuality. Either way, the cliché exists because fetishes are, indeed, incredibly common. According to the *Journal of Sex Research*, one in six people report engaging in some form of fetish play . . . and at last count, over five hundred distinct fetishes have been identified![12]

Many fetishists can identify a specific moment, often in childhood or early adolescence, when their specific object(s) became connected with feelings of arousal and desire. These BDSM origin stories often represent formative moments in their understanding of who and what they are, and new research indicates that this might be just one aspect of a far broader difference in how these folks experience the world around them! A recent study of self-identified objectophiles (people who experience both sexual desire and romantic love for inanimate objects) found that they are significantly more likely to report a prior diagnosis of autism spectrum disorders *and* consistent-over-time synesthesia, a neurological condition in which the brain forms associations between unrelated things, such as "hearing" color, "smelling" words, or ascribing anthropomorphic personality traits to inanimate objects.[13]

Regardless of whether someone has a fetish for a particular object because they associate it with a pleasurable memory from their past, it is consistently portrayed as sexy within their culture, or they are simply wired to attribute desirable traits to usually common objects, the simple fact is that object desires are incredibly common, deeply personal, and represent a positive perception of what the object symbolizes for them rather than a deficit that exists somewhere else in the fetishist's life or relationships. Or, as artist Dasha Yildirim puts it, "People love objects because they reflect what we value in ourselves."[14]

TRANSFORMATIONS: For a small subset of kinky people, the idea of transforming or of being transformed is profoundly erotic. They might have fantasies of growing or shrinking in size in ways that enhance their power-exchange desires. Being very small and having a giant dominant who overpowers or takes care of you is a popular theme among transformation fetishists. Likewise, sci-fi–inspired fantasies of being swallowed whole (vore) and enveloped into a warm, womb-like body turns many people on. These more "fantastical fantasies" can seem bizarre to those who don't share them, even among other kinksters. It's okay to not understand why someone finds the things they do sexy. What's not okay is shaming them for having harmless (if perhaps weird) desires. There is something really hot about weaving implausible story lines into our sexual scripts! When we remove the constraints of everyday reality from what we allow ourselves to fantasize about, we open up a whole new world of sensory and emotional possibility. We'll discuss this more in the next chapter when we look at the equally unlikely themes common in more socially acceptable forms of erotica.

Identity

As scary as it can be for us to realize that our partners fantasize about other people or situations that don't include us, it can be even more overwhelming to learn that they fantasize about being someone else entirely. When we learn that our partner daydreams about exploring new identities or even orientations, it can evoke a visceral reaction within us. After all, it was overwhelming enough to learn that they had interests and desires that were so very different from our own. The notion that they might fantasize about being someone else entirely can shake the foundations of who and what we understood them to be and cause us to question whether we are the person they want to be with. Some of the most common of these identity fantasies include . . .

GENDER FLUIDITY: We live in a golden age of gender-diversity awareness. Our scientific and popular understanding of sex and gender has expanded significantly due to increased genetic and neuroscience research as well as activists willing to share their own lived experiences of gender. This is a wonderful thing that only serves to make us kinder, more empathetic, and more aware of the lives and experiences of our friends, families, and neighbors. However, for many of us, this ever-expanding vocabulary of gender can be confusing, even threatening. We were raised with a binary understanding of male and female, man and woman. The XY and XX chromosomes were taught in middle-school science alongside four-square diagrams of the nineteenth-century Austrian biologist Gregor Mendel's pea shoots. The rapid advances in our scientific understanding of gender have left many of us wondering if what we knew even about ourselves is true. After all, if we can't trust our own eyes to differentiate something as (seemingly) constant and observable as gender, with its blue/pink, penis/vulva markers, what else are we getting wrong about the world?

This confusion and the mistrust that can result is exactly why we have to understand what sex and gender are in order to understand the nature of sexual desire. Brynn Tannehill, the author of *Everything You Ever Wanted to Know about Trans (But Were Afraid to Ask)*, summarizes it thusly:

> In very simplistic terms, sex is what's between your legs and gender is what's between your ears. Sex refers to physical characteristics, and gender relates to behavioral and psychological ones. This includes not just genitalia, but a whole host of physical factors such as chromosomes, genetics, and epigenetics. Gender is how we see ourselves; whether man, woman, neither, or somewhere in between. Transgender people are those whose sex and gender do not match.[15]

Gender expression, on the other hand, is how one chooses to outwardly express their gender through things like clothing, hairstyles, makeup, and mannerisms. These three traits—sex, gender, and gender expression—can be represented in a myriad of different ways, by many different people—and even by the same person, if they enjoy creative self-expression. This is really important information, because these facts lay the foundation for a key point in our conversation here:

Being trans is not a kink.

While there are many barriers to gathering accurate demographic information about gender-diverse folks, our best estimate is that approximately 0.3–0.5 percent of the worldwide population is transgender.[16] In the United States, there are roughly 1.4 million trans citizens. And sure, some trans people are also kinky! But their kink identity is a part of their sexual or relational expression that exists separately from their gender identity. It is 100 percent possible to be a vanilla trans person. In fact, a point of frustration for many trans- or gender-nonconforming folks is in the frequent fetishization they experience from nontrans (cisgender) people. Just like skin color, ethnicity, or body size, trans bodies are often sexualized in a way that can feel dehumanizing to the person being fetishized.

So, if being trans is not a kink; and if trans people, like people of color or people with larger bodies, do not want to be objectified based on their appearance; why are we discussing gender fluidity in this book? Because humans are novelty-seeking creatures who love variety. As a result, it is common for people of all genders to seek out erotic media that feature gender-diverse performers or spin tales of gender transformation. And when their partners discover that they've been exploring themes of gender fluidity, there can be stressed, worried reactions from both partners. One, discovering a new side to their partner, may wonder if, perhaps, their partner is seeking out these themes because they identify as trans and are holding back a secret desire to adjust their gender identity or presentation in some way. This concern can leave the partner feeling afraid that if their partner wants to transition (in some as-yet-uncertain way), they might be left behind, cast aside as a poor fit for their beloved's new identity. For the partner exploring, there can be many fears that sharing these desires and thoughts with their partner could bring up. Some, who are not trans, may fear that their kink being misrepresented could cause their partner to make assumptions that aren't true. For others, who may be considering transition, it can lead to the fear that their partner might not accept their newfound trans identity.

It is important to note here that for some (certainly not all) trans people, the BDSM community's acceptance of diverse genders and incorporation of notions of gender during play can provide the first safe space some people have to experiment with a different notion of gender than the one they are assigned at birth. We've already said (though it bears repeating) that being trans is not a kink. For those who find their identity through kinky play, there tends to be a shift (though not universally by any stretch) away from feminization as a form of BDSM as it becomes apparent that these moments evoke a sense of euphoria rather than the elements of shame and degradation that are usually incorporated into these types of scenes. And while trans experiences with gender play are important, the vast majority of people engaging in these types of play are not "eggs" (trans people who have not yet realized they want to transition). In fact, "gender-bending" was identified in Lehmiller's research as the seventh most common fantasy.[17]

There are kinks and fetishes that center around playing with gender presentation, such as cross-dressing (wearing clothing associated with the gender opposite of the wearers for arousal or sensory purposes), sissification/dollification (the use of extremely stereotypical feminine apparel/behavior as a way to humiliate the wearer), and bimbofication/himbofication (the use of extremely gender-stereotyped clothing as a way to hypersexualize the wearer), but none of these practices are intended to represent the wearer's authentic gender or sexual identity. They are exaggerations intended to tease, arouse, degrade, or enhance—but never to define. It is entirely possible to play with ideas of gender within our relationships, sexual expressions, and solo fantasies without having this play carry over into our understanding of our own core gender identities.

SAME-SEX IMAGERY: As we've come to see, variety is the spice of life and the human mind is an infinitely creative source of inspiration. It should not be surprising to learn that many folks who identify as "exclusively straight" (59 percent of heterosexual women and 26 percent of heterosexual men) report fantasizing about sex with someone of the same gender.[18] Polyamory, open relationships, and BDSM/kink are not topics taught in high-school sex-ed class—or even in many college-level human sexuality courses—and when they show up in popular media, it's often as the butt of a joke or as a warning sign of danger. Because of this, homosexuality is the primary form of sexual difference that we feel both familiar with and curious about. This is also true for folks who identify as LGBTQIA+ (curiosity about heterosexuality), but it tends to occur less frequently than it does for heterosexuals. This might be because many queer-identifying people *have* had experiences with opposite-gender partners at one point or another, and so they don't report the same degree of curiosity that we see in heterosexual folks.

Researchers who study sexual desires have identified four main types of same-sex fantasy:

1. Brief, general fantasies about unexpected forms of sexual orientation

2. More detailed fantasies about complicated expressions of erotic orientation

3. Fantasies . . . "by heterosexual males who enjoy the thought of lesbianism"[19]

4. Straight men who fantasize about what it would be like to have sex with other men . . . in the context of a threesome with a woman[20]

In other words, the desire to experience what sex and intimacy might be like with a partner of the opposite (or different) gender from themselves is incredibly common and only occasionally representative of our primary sexual orientation. What do I mean by "primary" sexual orientation? Like gender identity, sexual orientation can be far less binary than we might expect. Sexologist Alfred Kinsey created his famous six-point scale (developed in a time before the terms bi- and pansexual were common) to help visualize the spectrum of desire that he heard from his research participants:

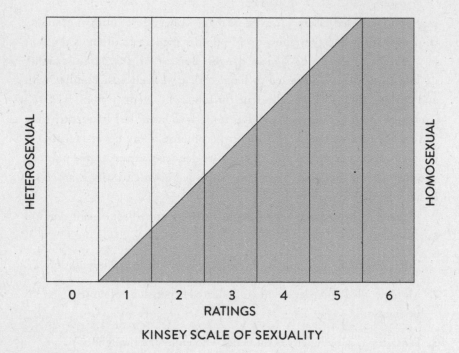

HETEROSEXUAL

HOMOSEXUAL

0   1   2   3   4   5   6

RATINGS

KINSEY SCALE OF SEXUALITY

Rating Description 0—Exclusively heterosexual (meaning "experiencing different gender attraction") 1—Predominantly heterosexual, only incidentally homosexual 2—Predominantly heterosexual, but more than incidentally homosexual 3—Equally heterosexual and homosexual 4—Predominantly homosexual, but more than incidentally heterosexual 5—Predominantly homosexual, only incidentally heterosexual 6—Exclusively homosexual (meaning "experiencing same gender attraction")[21]

This idea of identity spectrums carries over beyond our sexual orientation and gender identity! In my own work, I have created a tool called the Gender, Sexuality, and Relationship Diversity (GSRD) Carousel, which helps my clients visualize the variety of sexual and relational identities that we each contain. It can be a fascinating exercise to mark where you and your partner(s) each "sit" on the various wedges of the carousel (you can sit on a line between options too!) and then compare notes. It's a simple activity that can help you both better understand the nature of same-gender fantasies while leading to some powerful conversations about yourselves and your relationship.

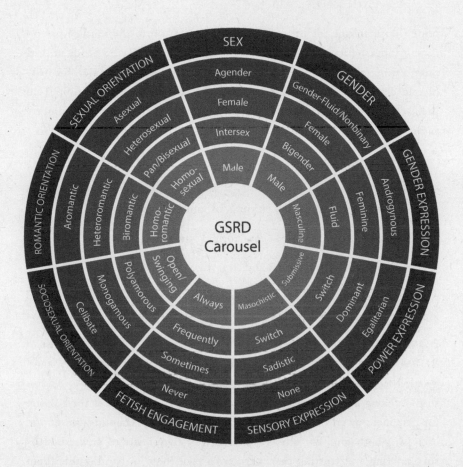

GENDER, SEXUALITY, AND RELATIONSHIP DIVERSITY CAROUSEL

Mark where you "sit" on each wedge of the wheel and ask your partner to do the same. Discuss where your positions complement one another or where there might be tension. And know that your seat in each wedge can (and might!) change over time.

There are times when our partner's sexual or relational orientation does not align with our own. These are usually called "mixed-orientation marriages" and are beyond the scope of this book. Like mixed kink/vanilla relationships, these are sometimes entered into consciously with full disclosure about their preferences from the LGBTQIA+ (or kinky) partner to their spouse. Perhaps more commonly, the partner who identifies as a sexual minority does not share this information either out of fear of rejection or hope that marriage might somehow change them into the kind of person their spouse believes them already to be. Researchers who study mixed-orientation relationships have identified several key rationales for why people choose to marry someone of a different sexual orientation from themselves, many of which resonate with kink-identified people who marry vanilla partners. These include marrying . . .

- at a young age, before their sexual identity has been able to fully crystalize

- in order to fulfill social, cultural, or familial expectations

- because it is the "natural" or "normal" next step in life

- in order to have children and a family

Most commonly *and* most importantly, both LGBTQIA+ persons and kinky people report marrying because they *genuinely love their spouse*.[22]

DOMINANCE AND SUBMISSION: Perhaps the most common form of BDSM play, and therefore the one that most folks feel they understand, dominance and submission allows the partners involved to create a relationship (lifelong or temporary) that gives them room to express their desire for personal power. For some (dominants), this means claiming power and exercising authority. For others (submissives), they relate to power best by surrendering and trusting their partner to take them in hand, guide them, and create a space for them to be free from the oppressive need to decide.[23] It is a common misconception that people who are dominant in the boardroom prefer to submit in the bedroom. In actuality, researchers have found that dominant personalities tend to be dominant in all areas of their lives. Submissives, on the other hand, often move between the need to claim and hold authority in some aspects of their lives (career, for example, or parenting) while ceding authority to their partners in the bedroom or in their relationships. "Switches" enjoy playing on both sides of the power-exchange slash, depending upon their mood or their partner. Many who consider themselves happily vanilla still enjoy playing with ideas of power in the bedroom; giving or taking orders, teasing and denial, and edging rather than evoking an orgasm are all forms of D/s play.

OTHER PERSONAS: In Jungian psychology, therapists work with the idea of archetypes: "Universal, inborn models of people, behaviors, or personalities that play a role in influencing human behavior."[24] Some of these are quite familiar even to nonclinicians, because they are present in the movies we watch and the fairy tales we read to our children at bedtime. The Ruler, the Lover, the Jester, the Magician—all are personas that we seem to innately understand because they are present in the tales told in every culture across time. Modern Jungian psychotherapists continue to identify archetypes that they use to help their clients better understand their feelings and relationships. Included among these are a variety of personas that Jungian practitioners recognize as being particularly "eros-inhibiting"[25] for those who have fallen into the behavior patterns they represent. Among these are the Pleaser, the Provider, the Dutiful Wife, the Responsible Mother, the Good Father, and the Disciplinarian. I suspect that these terms don't require much explanation; we intuitively know what they mean because they are so universal in nature. But I can almost hear you asking, "What on earth does this have to do with BDSM?" Well, for some kinksters . . . everything.

A number of subcultures within the BDSM community use role-play as their primary form of power exchange. Some forms of kinky role-play (or relationship dynamic) can look quite startling to the nonkinky observer—including, perhaps especially, age-play and pet-play. In age-play, the bottoming or submissive partner assumes the role of a younger, more childlike persona. This can range from role-playing as an infant (commonly referred to as ABDL, or "adult baby/diaper lover"); to role-playing as a snarky, bratty teenager; and every stage in between. Their topping/dominant partner assumes the role of caregiver (sometimes a governess/babysitter or sometimes a parental figure), one who provides both a space to indulge in play enjoyed by their childlike persona (coloring, watching cartoons, playing with toys, drinking from a bottle) and discipline and sensory play such as spanking. **This type of play is not an indicator that the folks involved are sexually interested in children.** Age-players are not interested in any kind of relationship with a child. They are sexually and romantically attracted to adults. They simply enjoy role-playing in a way that lets them explore and express their own internal childlike or protective archetypes. In the same way,

people who enjoy pet-play are in no way, shape, or form sexually attracted to animals. But they derive great pleasure from having a space to role-play the animal that personifies the qualities they wish to explore: the rambunctious freedom of a puppy; the dignity and refinement of a dressage pony; the indulged pampering of a kitten; the messy, gluttonous pig. Pet-players and their handler-tops tend to enjoy physical expressions of affection in their role-play: wrestling, crawling, petting, hair-brushing, massages, and so forth. Jungian therapist Chelsea Wakefield writes, "Many problems in life can be reduced to a failure of imagination. We get stuck in scripts and stories that are too small for the vastness of our souls. We live in boxes and constructs that limit our creative capacity and potential for fulfillment."[26] BDSM role players reject this paradigm and instead put their energy into creating a fantasy scene that allows for the exploration of other identities, the meeting of needs that they might not be able to express in their everyday lives, the setting down of adult (or even human) responsibilities, and the ability to simply *play* for a time. It is an outward expression of the myriad of archetypes and personas that make up each and every one of us and that so many of us are trained to put aside and ignore once we cross out of the "playing pretend" days of our youth.

Processing Discovery

My knowledge of BDSM and kink was very little to none. With my religious beliefs as a Mormon, I would have associated BDSM with darkness and evil. I would have thought kinks were for perverts. I had heard of sadomasochism, but the idea was very vague in my mind—a sexual perversion. [Finding out I had married someone who was into BDSM] was a little bit mind-blowing, to be honest. It was really hard, coming from such a sheltered background as I did. I don't want to say trauma—a little bit, maybe—but it was in a way. I understand why, now, but at the time, it was a huge breach of trust because I knew nothing about this before we got married. I understand why now, but at the time, it was confusing and scary because I associated it with darkness and evil.

He promised me he would not do it again, acknowledging that if it were me doing it, he would feel the same; that he would be uncomfortable and it would not be attractive. He could not make it go away, and I saw remnants of it in our closet when I looked under some clothes. He was hiding things from me. So I threw them out into the middle of the entryway, and he saw them when he got home from work. He told me that he had something like an "addiction" and said he was going to go to therapy. I remember being so excited thinking that my life is going to get better now because he was going to be "cured" and that we would have a "normal, healthy, sex life."

The way I describe it is that half of my brain understood it and had empathy and really wanted to support him. The other half was "no way. I did not sign up for this." I used to feel terrified. Now I can say, "It's not my thing, but it's his, and that's okay." I could not say that before. In the past I thought it was something to be controlled and exorcized (not literally). It brings up feelings of pride for how far I've come and how far he has come as well. But also sadness at how much was lost by trying to make it go away.

As far as my feelings toward BDSM/kink now? My feelings are positive, despite my lack of interest in it. I get very protective of people in the kink community when others negatively comment about them, call them perverts, weirdos, etc.

—Holly, 51

DOES THIS MEAN I'M NOT ENOUGH?

"If I looked more like the people in the videos she watches, she'd love me more."

"If he's into this stuff, he can't possibly be happy without it."

"If that's what they want—they can't want me."

If is a powerful word. It helps us to form connections in the brain between what is real and what is possible. In computer sciences, the if-then format is called a conditional statement and is used to tell the computer what action should follow a particular user choice. In classical logic, these if-then conditions are the backbone of deductive reasoning. Students spend hours learning how to differentiate between true and false assumptions based on various if-then scenarios. Our brains are wired to make these logical snap judgments and do so hundreds, if not thousands, of times per day. The problem is that our brains are wonderfully complex, incredibly intricate, and woefully stupid organs.

Our brains believe whatever we tell them. The more they hear something, the truer it becomes within the brain. That's why positive affirmations work. "There is MRI evidence suggesting that certain neural pathways are increased when people practice self-affirmation tasks. If you want to be super specific, the ventromedial prefrontal cortex—involved in positive valuation and self-related information processing—becomes more active when we consider our personal values."[27] Likewise, the placebo effect has been shown to work time and time again due in large part to our brain's suggestibility. "How placebos work is still not quite understood, but it involves a complex neurobiological reaction that includes everything from increases in feel-good neurotransmitters, like endorphins and dopamine, to greater activity in certain brain regions linked to moods, emotional reactions, and self-awareness. All of it can have therapeutic benefits."[28] It can also cause a lot of stress, fear, and anxiety when we do not recognize the power of the "ifs" we're creating for ourselves.

This is especially true and particularly insidious when it comes to sex. Madeleine Castellanos explains that

> When it comes to sexual desire, the brain can actually learn not to want sex for various reasons. Maybe you don't get as much enjoyment out of it compared to how much effort you put into it. Perhaps there has been pain or discomfort, and now your mind is trying to avoid experiencing that discomfort again. Positive or negative expectations can influence an experience by either enhancing it, ruining it, or anything in between. Depending on what you are expecting, you either open your mind up to an experience or shut yourself off from it.[29]

One of the ways that our brain's ability to experience pleasure can be influenced is through the reactions we have to and the judgments we form about our partner's kinks, fetishes, and other desires. When the message our brain receives is a steady stream of negative if-then statements, we can quickly lose our sense of connection not only to our partner but to our own sexual selves. It is impossible to separate our physiology from our emotions, thoughts, and relationship patterns. Our brains experience and respond to each of these "if" scenarios and use them to weave an interconnected "then" tapestry of identity and sensuality that is as physical as it is emotional or relational. Just a few of the variables that influence our sexual selves are . . .

Physiological Variables

- hormone levels

- thyroid functioning

- chronic pain/illness

- lack of sleep

- circulation or blood pressure issues

- neurological differences

- masturbation habits

- erectile and/or vaginal lubrication difficulties

- pelvic floor dysfunctions

- smell/taste of the body (ours and our partners)

Emotional Variables

- stress/anxiety

- anger/hurt

- sadness/depression

- fear/trauma

- disappointment

- pressure

- guilt/shame

- self-consciousness/body image concerns

- internal thoughts about sex and intimacy

- distraction, disconnection, dissociation (the three D's)

Social Variables

- childhood lessons about sex and relationships

- cultural expectations about sexuality and gender roles

- peer opinions about what is sexy/desirable

- ideas about what marriage/relationships "should" look like

- religious messages around sex, gender roles, and relationships

- media representation of sex and relationships

Relational Variables

- positive or negative feelings toward partner

- routine acts of kindness

- chore-sharing, parenting, and division of labor

- pressure to conceive or prevent pregnancy

- unspoken expectations

- unresolved conflicts and resentments

- making partner responsible for our pleasure

Use this chart to identify your personal libido influencers—both the things you notice turn you on and those moments or actions that turn you off.

BODY INFLUENCERS:	RELATIONSHIP INFLUENCERS:
SOCIAL INFLUENCERS:	CULTURAL INFLUENCERS:

Libido Changes

As you can see, our libido (or our sexual appetite) is influenced by a huge number of factors—some that we can control, many that we can't. When we get caught up in a mental cycle of if-then thoughts about our partner's kinks, it can quickly create a problem that goes beyond the emotional challenge of absorbing this new information and begins to manifest physically. When we are feeling stressed, anxious, or upset, decreased interest in sex and difficulty experiencing arousal is one of the biggest ways our body expresses these emotions. This is true for both partners—the one who is sitting with the stress and fear of discovery and/or the concurrent anxiety about possible rejection and the person who learns something new about their partner that leaves them afraid that there might be other secrets out there and anxious about what this new knowledge means for their relationship. This can create a vicious pattern that looks something like this:

KINKY PARTNER'S PATH TO LIBIDO LOSS

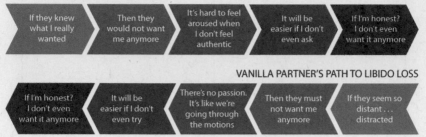

| If they knew what I really wanted | Then they would not want me anymore | It's hard to feel aroused when I don't feel authentic | It will be easier if I don't even ask | If I'm honest? I don't even want it anymore |

VANILLA PARTNER'S PATH TO LIBIDO LOSS

| If I'm honest? I don't even want it anymore | It will be easier if I don't even try | There's no passion. It's like we're going through the motions | Then they must not want me anymore | If they seem so distant... distracted |

PATH TO LIBIDO LOSS

As you can see, often this dynamic results in a "two ships passing in the night" paradigm that can be profoundly detrimental to our ability to connect sexually with each other.

This is not to say that all libido differences can be attributed to the thought patterns we've created for ourselves about our partner's desires. People can and do have variations in their natural sexual desire levels, which can often be challenging to navigate in a relationship. In fact, one of the leading issues that brings couples to counseling and specifically sex therapy is mismatched libido. Part of the problem is what Laurie Mintz calls "the pleasure gap"—the differences between genders in their experience of sexual pleasure and orgasms.[30] Mintz writes that among heterosexual partners, even where there is no vanilla-kink mismatch, only 64 percent of women reported having an orgasm during their last sexual encounter, compared to 91 percent of men.[31] The pleasure gap can feed into thought patterns that then negatively impact our libido. When we don't experience pleasure in our routine sexual encounters, we're less likely to expect pleasure from sex, which triggers the same negative thought cycle that can sever our brain's if-then connection of "If I have sex, then I will feel good." This in turn can impact our physiological libido levels and make us want sex less in general.[32] This is part of why healthy communication with our partner about pleasure (see chapters 4 and 5) and how we like to give and receive pleasure is so crucial to our experience of healthy libido and sexual satisfaction.

Desire Differences

A mismatched or shifting libido level isn't the only reason why partners in kinky-vanilla relationships can struggle with intimacy. It's quite possible for both partners to have a healthy libido and an active sex life together and still experience these moments in a way that feels painful or inadequate. Even in relationships where everything else aligns (people feel physically healthy, emotionally connected, personally desirous, and aren't carrying the negative thought patterns or social lessons that can get in the way of a vibrant, connected sex life with our partners) the vanilla-kink misalignment can present a challenge. Advice columnist Dan Savage coined the term "GGG—good, giving, and game" in the late 1990s as shorthand for what he suggests is reasonable to expect from a healthy partnership. "As Savage has explained: 'Think good in bed, giving based on a partner's sexual interests, and game for anything—within reason.'"[33] The term has grown in popularity since Savage introduced it to the world, and it's now quite common to see the acronym GGG used in dating profiles as well as sex and relationship writings both within the mainstream and BDSM/kink communities.

Most of us enjoy sex and are genuinely invested in our partner's happiness, which makes it easy to be GGG for our partners organically. For others, the "good, giving, and game" descriptor is weaponized against them, either internally (through a misinterpretation of "good" to mean valuable, worthy, or obedient) or externally by folks who use coercive tactics such as pleading, guilt trips, passive aggressiveness, and emotional withholding in order to convince their partners that setting a boundary means that they aren't willing to "give" them what they want.

One of the most difficult challenges is when someone is genuinely willing to be "good, giving, and game" and to push their personal comfort zones a bit in order to indulge their partner's desires . . . and still finds themselves feeling uncomfortable and/or unaroused. It's not a matter of feeling pressured to perform in the moment; they may be eager to experiment or to meet their partner's request. But in the moment they simply . . . aren't into it—at all. They may even realize they're having a viscerally negative reaction to the requested activity. *That's okay!* It's always acceptable to realize that something just isn't working for you. When this happens to one or both partners and we fail to honor our feelings, pause, and regroup or make a change, we can inadvertently trigger a negative feedback loop of . . .

Desire/Distaste -> Discomfort -> Disconnection -> Disappointment

When we talk about the idea of being "good, giving, and game," the goal is not to be giving to the point of self-denial! Particularly not when our willingness to give to our partner causes a strongly negative reaction for ourselves. Sex should never mean suffering. In any relationship negotiation, whether we're talking about doing the dishes or trying something new in the bedroom, there is often a *yes* partner (the one who desires the behavior) and a *no* partner (the one who would rather not). We tend to view these experiences as separate and distinct, but really they function more like an intersecting ebb and flow of emotion, with each person having moments of shared pain and compassion while approaching the conflict from opposing perspectives.

NO PARTNER **YES PARTNER**

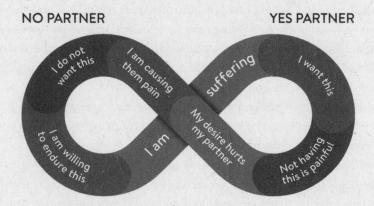

EMOTIONAL FEEDBACK LOOP

This emotional feedback loop is not limited to partners trying to navigate kink-vanilla desire differences. One of the most common concerns expressed by my female clients is worries related to body image and self-esteem. Let's use a fictional scenario, based on some of the most common challenges that bring couples to sex therapy, to take a closer look at how this feedback loop can play out in a relationship when one partner looks at the other and says, "You know what I want right now? I want to watch you on top of me":

Lida has been looking forward to date night all week. She showers and shaves using the body wash Dylan bought her for their last anniversary. It's the same scent as her perfume, and she loves the way it makes her feel when she wears it: confident and sexy. After drying her hair, Lida adds just a touch of tinted moisturizer, mascara, and a swipe of rose-tinted lip balm to her face. She's never felt comfortable being all dolled up, but a little touch of color is nice. She slips into the dress and stands in the mirror, admiring what it does for her. Lida has always felt a little embarrassed about the curve of her tummy. She grew up with fashion models and fitness influencers setting the standard, and Lida just . . . never felt like she matches up. This dress hides her belly (and the stretch marks that adorn it) beneath a stylish ruching detail. She feels beautiful. She closes the bedroom door behind her as she goes to meet Dylan, who is waiting for her in the car.

Dinner is lovely. They have a handful of favorite restaurants, and this is one of them. Lida orders the same thing she always gets. It's her favorite and she likes knowing she won't be disappointed if she orders it again. Dessert comes and goes and eventually the server leaves them alone to chat over their glasses of wine. The corners of Dylan's eyes crinkle when they smile in a way that Lida finds captivating. She asks what Dylan is thinking about. "I'm thinking about tonight, about being alone with you. I'm thinking about how much I want you." Lida blushes. They've been together for years, but Dylan is still able to bring the color to her cheeks. She smiles back. "What do you want?"

"You know what I want right now?" whispers Dylan, leaning in over their now-empty wine glasses. (**I Want This**) "I want to watch you on top of me." Lida's smile falters just briefly before she catches herself. She hopes Dylan didn't notice. She can read the excitement in Dylan as they make their way to the car. What had been an evening of excited anticipation now feels like dread. (**I Do Not Want This**) Lida keeps thinking about her stomach. The way it rolls when she's sitting. The pink, purple, and silver stretch marks that she can't seem to get rid of no matter how much cocoa butter she uses. The way her breasts seem so small compared to her belly. She can't stop thinking about it. It's such a little thing, though, and it will make Dylan so happy. They never ask for something specific like this. She has no reason to say no. She's terrified.

Dylan leads her back to the bedroom. The mirror feels like an enemy now. The dress falls to the floor as Lida reaches for the light switch. "Leave it on," whispers Dylan. "I want to see you." Lida is grateful that Dylan can't see her flinch when she hears those words. She pushes the anxiety to the back of her mind as they tumble into bed. This is the part she loves: the kissing, the feel of skin on skin, how intensely *safe* she feels wrapped in Dylan's arms. They move together, Dylan above her, smiling. They roll and suddenly she finds herself astride Dylan's hips. As much as she tries not to, Lida can feel her body react as she becomes aware just how bright the ceiling light is, how exposed she feels, how intently Dylan is watching her. She feels tense, embarrassed. She resists the urge to cover herself with her hands and closes her eyes to avoid Dylan's gaze. (**I Am Willing to Endure This Pain**) "It's such a little thing," she tells herself. Lida's discomfort is not worth sacrificing Dylan's pleasure. She tries to pretend she's somewhere else or at least that the lights are off. It feels like she can physically *feel* Dylan watching her as she moves. She was having such a lovely time . . . now she wishes she were anywhere but here.

Dylan reaches up to caress Lida's shoulders, running their hands down the length of her arms and grasping her hands, aware of the change in Lida's movements and facial expression. She no longer seems connected. Dylan feels the tension in her muscles, the way she clings to Dylan's hands. She is so beautiful. They have been thinking about this, planning this night, for weeks. Dylan has daydreamed about the look on Lida's face as she moves on top of them. The bounce and sway of her breasts. The soft feel of her hips as Dylan holds and guides them. This is nothing like that.

(**My Desire Hurts My Partner**) Dylan and Lida have been together for a really long time. They've seen each other through the celebrations and crises. Dylan knows what a happy Lida looks like, and this isn't it. This dawning awareness pulls Dylan out of the moment they'd anticipated for so long. They can see Lida's gritted teeth. They know she would never say a word about how uncomfortable she feels right now. But beneath her closed eyelids? Dylan worries that they can see tears. They pull Lida down beside them and wrap their arms around her. Dylan kisses her forehead and says, "Let's just hold each other for a bit." (**Not Having This Is Painful**) Dylan would never vocalize this to Lida, but the disappointment is crushing. Dylan is a highly visual person and finds Lida incredibly sexy. Now? They feel guilty for asking something from her that has caused her such distress. Dylan fears that the next time they go to fantasize about

Lida on top of them that they will feel guilty rather than aroused. They don't want to think about her discomfort and shame in that moment. (**I Am Willing to Endure This Pain**) Dylan decides that they will just try to put this particular fantasy out of their mind. It's been a favorite fantasy, and they genuinely love the way Lida looks in these moments, but Dylan's pleasure isn't worth Lida's pain. (**I Am Suffering**) Dylan feels like they've ruined the evening by asking Lida to fulfill their fantasy. Lida knows Dylan just as well as they know her. She can feel Dylan's disappointment. They never stop in the middle of sex like this. She feels like she let them down, like she let her own discomfort ruin their evening. Lida and Dylan kiss and stroke each other. After a few minutes, they regroup, turn off the lights, and return to making love. Shortly after Lida orgasms, Dylan does too. They fall asleep wrapped in each other's arms. Both fall asleep thinking to themselves, "This could have been so much better."

Situations like these happen every day and in every kind of relationship. Whether it's trying a new sexual position, experimenting with a blindfold, or receiving a sound spanking, there are inevitably going to be times when our partner wants something that we don't. And that's okay! As we learned from our conversation about the libido, being aware of what we think and how we feel about a given situation can be key to successful intimacy. When we honor our partner with the truth of where we are mentally and emotionally, and trust them to be open to creative compromise, we can set boundaries for ourselves that actually promote *more* intimacy rather than shutting it down. While it sounds counterintuitive, the key to hot, passionate sex and deep, meaningful connection often lies in our ability to say no.

BUILDING FENCES, NOT WALLS

Social scientists have conducted many experiments to understand how people use and move through various spaces. In one of my favorite "tales of cool science," they hosted parties on the rooftops of several high-rise buildings and observed how their guests interacted with one another and with the space. They found that when the party was held on a rooftop that lacked railings or some other barrier around the edges of the building, the people stayed close together and tended to congregate in the center of the roof space. They stayed far away from the edges—much farther than was actually necessary in order to safely move around the party. On the other hand, when the researchers hosted their science-parties on the roofs of buildings that did feature a guard-rail? Their guests spread out much more and used the entirety of the roof's expanse. Many even went right up to the edges they'd taken such pains to avoid before and looked down to see how high they were. The conclusion we can draw from these experiments is that boundaries are not just tools to keep us out of danger but they also help us recognize where we will be safe. When we understand the safe zones? We go a bit further than we would without the boundary there.

I talk about these experiments with most of my clients. I believe that boundary setting is one of the most important tasks we can accomplish in therapy, but I want the folks I work with to see this process not as excluding what we don't want but rather of articulating what we do. We see this process in action when we take children to a playground. Most playgrounds these days have fences around them. The fences are low, typically, and often made of a material that we can see through, such as chain link. They have openings in them so that people can pass through as they enter or leave. Fences define without excluding. Often we tell our children, "Stay inside the fence and you can play on anything you want."

Researchers who study environmental design have found that humans have different reactions to different kinds of physical barriers. When a given amount of space is enclosed within a fence that allows us to see what's on the other side, it feels expansive and spacious to us. On the other hand, when walls exist, particularly high walls, we tend to feel enclosed and constrained—even if there is no difference in the amount of space actually available. Researchers drew three conclusions from their experiments:

1. The most important function an environment can provide for its inhabitants is safety.

2. Among other things, safety depends on how far and how easily one can sense or move through an environment.

3. Permeable boundaries should make spaces feel less enclosed. The reasoning is that the more permeable a boundary, the more an

environment will be visible. Increased visibility means less danger; and because perceived enclosure is a proxy for danger, the more permeable a boundary, the less enclosed a space should seem.[34]

In other words, people feel safest when they have clearly defined boundaries that let them see what's on the other side. Fences, not walls.

What, you may be wondering, do environmental design and rooftop social experiments have to do with setting boundaries around sex and intimacy in relationships? Strangely enough, everything. The key to effective boundary setting is to understand that your boundaries can only ever apply to *you*. It is impossible, and I would argue unethical, to try to impose boundaries on another person. Our power lies in the decisions we make for and about ourselves. We cannot *make* anyone do anything. We can *ask* our partners for anything, however reasonable or unreasonable the request may be, and then make our own choices based on the answer we receive. The more we are able to define our boundaries as fences rather than walls, defining what we find acceptable rather than listing the behaviors that we object to, the more likely our partners are to perceive these boundaries as expansive rather than constraining. In other words, figuring out where you can say yes is a highly effective way to define your no.

At the end of this book, you will find the Sprinkles Fence Building Chart. Your answers are not meant to be a contract with or a promise to your partner. Rather, the chart is a tool for you to start to sort out the disparate practices and play that fall under the umbrella of BDSM and to create a space for you to reflect on where your fences are. For each activity, you can express curiosity, desire, open-mindedness, trust, reflectiveness, and boundaries. There are no right or wrong answers, and your feelings about a given category might change over time. That's okay! This is one tool out of many that you can use to begin to consider where your personal fences are, right now.

Fields Within Fences

In the same way that finding our yeses can help us more clearly define what we don't want, our partner's fantasies and fetishes shouldn't be taken as a statement on the desire they feel for us. It is possible to find multiple wildly different types of people or play sexy, and we are already one of their yeses!

Likewise, if we take the time to consider the themes of our own fantasies (something we're going to spend more time doing in the next chapter), we often realize that there's a surprising amount of variety there as well. Moving forward, we will turn our attention away from focusing on understanding the differences between ourselves and our partners and begin to put our energy into creating a field of common themes and desires. When we can meet each other in a creative space of mutual yeses, clearly bound by the hard limits that define our space, magic can happen. I'll meet you there.

MORE TO READ ON THIS TOPIC

Attached: The New Science of Adult Attachment and How It Can Help You Find—and Keep—Love

Amir Levine and Rachel Heller

Pleasure Activism: The Politics of Feeling Good

adrienne maree brown

Sex Smart: How Your Childhood Shaped Your Sexual Life and What to Do About It: Transform Your Sex Life

Aline P. Zoldbrod

4

Finding Your Sprinkles

I still remember the first romance novel I ever read. I found it at the grocery store the summer between fifth and sixth grade, where I threw it on the conveyor belt while my mother was distracted. It was titled *Banner O'Brien* and centered around a young woman who earned her medical degree in the late 1800s before traveling west to work with an arrogant and entitled male doctor. They butt heads with each other. She rebels against him, and he overcomes her protestations. They fall in love, of course. I was captivated. The next novel I managed to sneak under my parents' noses was Johanna Lindsey's *Silver Angel*, which featured an aristocratic young woman who is captured and trafficked into sexual slavery as a haram concubine. There she encounters the arrogant and entitled Pasha, her ostensible owner. They fight. She resists. He overpowers. They fall in love. Are you sensing a theme?

The novels of Kathleen E. Woodiwiss are filled with scenarios in which the characters find themselves caught up in power dynamics that evolve into erotic relationships. In middle school, my friend Sarah and I would pass these novels back and forth between classes, writing each other notes in the margins highlighting particularly witty retorts from the heroine or exceptionally erotic gestures from her antagonist-slash-soulmate. Woodiwiss revolutionized the bodice-ripper genre. Her plots ranged from penniless orphan fleeing from sexual assault being mistaken for a prostitute and kidnapped by handsome and ruthless ship's captain, to aristocratic woman married off to a suitable husband finds herself longing for the decidedly unsuitable visitor from abroad, to Saxon princess conquered by invading Normans finds herself falling in love with her Viking captor, to Southern belle disguised as a boy is rescued and protected from harm by a handsome Union officer. Romantic fiction novels make up nearly half of all paperbacks sold in North America; and unlike many of the novels from my youth, they are more diverse and inclusive than ever. Authors such as Jasmine Guillory, and Talia Hibbert are creating vibrant tales of love and lust that reflect their readership and highlight the many ways in which we can experience love and attraction. These books are read primarily by women (84 percent of readers) who are between eighteen and forty-four years old (53 percent of readers).[1] They are sold in every bookstore and market in the country and are considered a staple of modern publishing. Romance novels are not tawdry products sold in back rooms or in plain paper wrapping. They are an incredibly popular facet of mainstream pop culture, and yet nearly every plot point I described above is an overt story about power-exchange relationships and other elements of BDSM:

- The prisoner held against her will and forced to submit to the desires of a more powerful person? Bondage.

- The young professional trying to prove herself to the intimidating employer? Discipline.

- The proud military officer taking an isolated young boy under his protection? Dominance.

- A dutiful court lady married off to a man she does not love in order to protect her family name? Submission.

- The slave reduced in status and considered nothing more than sexual property? Sadomasochism.

We read tales of BDSM voraciously, but because the characters are wrapped in tartan and silk or flannel and denim rather than latex and leather, we think of their relationship dynamics as simply passionate, romantic, or . . . vanilla.

It makes sense that these tropes would pervade our fantasies about sex and romance. The human mind craves novelty, and, as a result, we fantasize about a variety of novel scenarios—even when we are, at that moment, having missionary-position sex with our partner in our own bedroom. Justin Lehmiller surveyed over four thousand people about their sexual fantasies and identified seven main themes, many of which we see explored throughout pop culture from erotic romance novels to classical art and PG-13 romantic comedies. These include:

1. Multi-partner sex (threesomes, orgies, gang bangs)

2. BDSM

3. Novelty, adventure, and variety (doing something that's new and different for you, such as a new position or setting)

4. Taboo sex acts (doing something that is socially or culturally forbidden)

5. Passion, romance, and intimacy (emotionally connecting with a partner or feeling loved, appreciated, or desired)

6. Being in a nonmonogamous relationship (swinging, polyamory, cuckolding, or having an open relationship)

7. Gender-bending and homoeroticism (pushing the boundaries of your gender identity/role/expression and/or sexual orientation)[2]

While the details may vary (hence the infinite variety of erotica available on the various hub and tube sites), the overarching themes are universal. These are experiences that we all daydream about. (Those of us who do daydream, anyway—not all of us do!) Some of us even live them out. The universality is important for us to know and recognize, because so many of us are raised with a sense of guilt, shame, and isolation when it comes to our sexual curiosities. Understanding just how common even the most niche desires can be, knowing that we are not alone for being turned on by whatever it is that turns us on, is a powerful force for healing. So, let's talk about what turns *you* on.

FLESHING OUT YOUR FANTASIES

People fantasize about all kinds of things, all day long. We daydream about our kids growing up and graduating from medical school. We imagine our obnoxious coworker getting tossed out the office window. We reminisce about the glory days of our senior prom or the big game. Sometimes we get lost imagining ourselves as astronauts or vampire hunters, emperors or house pets. Kalina Christoff, the founder of the Cognitive Neuroscience of Thought Laboratory at the University of British Columbia, explains that daydreaming opens us up to possibilities that the logical mind cannot pursue: "The power of the wandering mind is precisely the fact that it censors nothing. It can make connections you would never otherwise make." Daydreaming is an inherently creative process, Christoff says, because the daydreamer is open to bizarre new options. Fresh insights and methods that don't already exist in the larger culture are revealed through this solitary style of brain-work. By contrast, analytical thinking, logical thinking, is all about the exclusion and critiquing of ideas so that the brain can become a guided laser that operates with surgical precision. The conscious, analytical style of thinking that our schools train us to use always silences the bizarre or unpopular ideas that the daydreaming mind might try on.[3]

We can be mermaids or Mary, Queen of Scots, in our fantasies. We can exact our revenge on frustrating colleagues or seduce the boy we had a crush on back in college. All bets are off and every option is open when we daydream.

Our physical self will react to our mental and emotional state, and what we think about is directly connected to this reaction. When we are angry with that annoying colleague and imagine stapling their tie to their desk, we experience a rush of adrenaline and our blood pressure rises. When we remember a powerful moment from our romantic past or envision a scenario that we wish we could experience, our body responds accordingly. Our heart beats faster and our blood vessels dilate, which allows blood to flow to the genitals and cheeks, leaving us feeling flushed and tingly. Erectile tissue such as the nipples and genitals swell and become more sensitive. If you have a penis, it may get hard. If you have a vulva, it may become wet.

One fascinating point to keep in mind is that people do not necessarily fantasize in the same way. Most folks can create a mental image of their daydream scenario. A slightly smaller number are able to incorporate other sensations such as scent; if they imagine they are lying in a field of flowers, they can conjure up the scent in their mind. A small handful of people experience a phenomenon called aphantasia, the inability to create mental images or recall memories of what people or places in their lives look like.[4] I have frequently worked with couples with differences in imagination that prove frustrating. One partner sends a lengthy text, laying out in exquisite detail what they'd like to do to the other. They eagerly await the response. They can't wait to see in what direction their paramour will take the story. They feel that jolt of electric anticipation when they see the three pulsing dots that indicate a response is forthcoming. And then the crushing disappointment that hits them when they read, "Oh, that sounds nice." These moments begin with the best of intentions and the highest of hopes. The goal is to let their partner know that they are not only thinking of them in this moment but also desiring them. The benign response they receive in return falls flat and leaves them feeling awkward or rejected. When we unpack these moments together, what we usually realize is that their brains create fantasies in different ways. Once we recognize these differences, we can work with them.

I created the Fleshing Out Your Fantasies Worksheet to help my clients explore the details of their sensual fantasies. When I'm working with an individual, I give them a copy to take home and reflect on between sessions. Often this exercise is the first time they've ever paid attention to the recurring themes of their intimate mental world. After they've completed the worksheet, we discuss it together in session and explore their reactions to the answers. Many people experience guilt, shame, embarrassment, or confusion about their sensual fantasies. For some, this confusion is borne out of the fact that they may not fantasize at all! And that's okay! Some folks just aren't visual thinkers . . . they don't fantasize in images or stories. Others might have grown up in a family or a culture that warned us not to indulge in sexy thoughts. No matter what your experience with fantasy is, where you are right now is just fine.

Our work together is to explore these negative spaces, to identify what counts as a "normal" or "healthy" fantasy versus a "weird" or "unhealthy" fantasy, and to find ways for them to explore elements of their fantasies in ways that feel safe to them. When I'm working with couples, I give both partners two copies of the worksheet. I ask them to complete one for themselves and to try to anticipate their partner's responses with the other. Comparing these together in session and seeing how much they know about each other's daydreams can be an empowering and enlightening experience. You can download and print this worksheet at stefanigoerlich.com/with-sprinkles-on-top-worksheets.html#/.

Fleshing Out the Fantasy Worksheet

Ideally, I would like to have sex _____ times per _____ .

Ideally, I would like to masturbate _____ times per _____ .

I think about sex:

☐ Quite Often ☐ Sometimes

☐ Hardly Ever ☐ Rarely/Never

My favorite sexual position is _____ .

I enjoy this because it makes me feel . . .

Physically: _____ .

Mentally: _____ .

Emotionally: _____ .

During sex, I like to:

☐ Lead the action

☐ Let my partner lead

☐ Take turns leading

I daydream about having sex . . .

☐ Indoors ☐ In Public

☐ Outdoors ☐ In an Imaginary/Fantasy Place

☐ At Home ☐ In a Different Time (historical)

☐ At Work ☐ Other: _____

I daydream about having sex with . . .

☐ My partner ☐ Someone of my gender

☐ An Ex ☐ Multiple People

☐ A Stranger ☐ Others Watching

☐ Other: _____

I would rather:

☐ Seduce ☐ Be Seduced

☐ Force ☐ Be Forced

☐ Take Turns

I like to read/watch/imagine scenarios in which I feel . . .

☐ Helpless ☐ In Charge ☐ Connected

☐ Protected ☐ Ravished ☐ Naughty/Bad

☐ Cherished ☐ Degraded ☐ Beautiful

☐ Seduced ☐ Objectified ☐ Worshipped

☐ Other: _____

☐ Other: _____

I like to be called nicknames that make me feel . . .

☐ Cute (Girl/Boy, Princess, Kitten, Baby)

☐ Adored (Darling, Sweetheart, Love)

☐ Dirty (Slut, Whore, Cunt, Bitch)

☐ Powerful (Goddess, Master/Mistress, Sir/Ma'am, Boss)

☐ Other: _____

When I fantasize, I see the scene:

☐ Through my own eyes, experiencing everything in the scene firsthand

☐ Through another person's eyes in the scene, watching myself experience everything

☐ From outside everything, as if I were watching myself and others on a movie screen

☐ I don't visualize anything when I fantasize

☐ Other: _____

When I fantasize, I like to feel _____ by/to my partner:

☐ Beloved, like we're soulmates

☐ Connected, as if we love one another

☐ Casual, like a friend with benefits

☐ Anonymous, like a hookup with a stranger

☐ Objectified, like I'm my partner's toy

My fantasies sometimes involve . . .

☐ Gender swapping or being another gender

☐ Same-sex intimacy

☐ Androgyny or ambiguity around gender

☐ Partners who are alien, objects, or otherwise nonhuman

☐ Penetrating (if you have a vulva) or being penetrated (if you have a penis)

What are you usually wearing in your fantasies?

☐ Nothing at all ☐ Costumes or Uniforms

☐ Lingerie ☐ Corsets or other restrictive items

☐ Street Clothes ☐ Leather, Rubber, Latex, Chain, etc.

☐ Formal Attire ☐ Other: _____

What is your partner usually wearing in your fantasies?

☐ Nothing at all ☐ Costumes or Uniforms

☐ Lingerie ☐ Corsets or other restrictive items

☐ Street Clothes ☐ Leather, Rubber, Latex, Chain, etc.

☐ Formal Attire ☐ Other: _____

Sex for me is about:

☐ Intimacy ☐ Spirituality

☐ Romance ☐ Reproduction/Procreation

☐ Pleasure ☐ Sensation

☐ Play ☐ Conquest

☐ Power/Control ☐ Other: _____

When I daydream about sex, climax or orgasm:

☐ Happens for me ☐ Happens for my partner

☐ Happens for both of us ☐ Isn't an important part of the fantasy

If they were movies, most of my sexual fantasies would be rated:

☐ G ☐ PG ☐ PG-13

☐ R ☐ X ☐ XXX

What is your most common sexual daydream?

_____

_____

_____

_____

_____

_____

Is there a fantasy scenario you enjoy thinking about but find
shameful or embarrassing?

_____

_____

_____

_____

_____

If you could rewrite your last sexual encounter, what would you
change? Add?

_____

_____

_____

_____

_____

The really fun work starts after we have fleshed out the fantasy because now we have a personalized framework—or, as I like to think of it, a sandbox to play in. The creative process of sitting with your worksheet, and perhaps those of your partners, and brainstorming various scenarios that let you weave in as many "yes" elements as possible without stepping into any "no-thank-you" elements often results in conversations filled with laughter, thoughtfulness, and (if done properly) the delightful tension of building anticipation. One woman that I worked with used the worksheet to identify the following themes: She noticed that her favorite position was classic missionary because it accommodated her body-image anxiety. She liked to be able to control the progress of an encounter and to lead the way; yet at the same time, she enjoyed the feeling of being seduced. Upon reflection, she noticed that her fantasies were never explicit; she didn't focus on climax, and she and her partner were often very dressed up rather than nude or wearing lingerie. The most erotic elements of her daydreams were thoughts of having sex with her partner in public while others watched. She enjoyed this scenario because it left her feeling both playful and naughty, dirty, and adored. And she was absolutely certain that this was a scenario that she wanted to keep firmly in the realm of fantasy. As we unpacked her responses on the worksheet and played with various combinations, she came up with a number of ways to weave elements of her fantasies into their real-world intimacy. These included . . .

- Checking into the upper floor of a hotel and having sex with the curtains open, as the sun sets. This scenario, when enacted with the room lights off, allows her to have that thrill of "What if we get caught?" without violating the consent of people passing below them.

- Dressing up and going out to dinner, with seats at separate tables across the restaurant. Partner periodically sending text messages or sending notes via the waiter that alternate between "You look so lovely" and "I can't wait to use and defile you." Playing with the incongruence between her desires to be seduced and dirtied.

- Masturbating in their bedroom while her partner listened to her from outside their door. Alternately, recording a voice memo of her masturbating and sending it to him to listen to on his own. These scenarios accommodate her concerns about body image while allowing her to experience a sense of being watched/observed in a safe and controlled way.

- Her partner coming home from work in his business suit and then setting up a video camera, which he tells her is live streaming, then asking her to give him a lap dance for their audience. Being allowed to take the lead, determine what clothing she would remove and when, which parts of her body she would expose and how, while imagining that this whole encounter was being watched by an audience of hundreds was a very appealing idea for her.

Each of these scenarios stayed well within her comfort zone and her fantasy life, and when her partner was presented with this list of options, they were met with great enthusiasm. This example uses just one individual's fantasy worksheet. When you complete it together with a partner, the possibilities for sexy, creative, mutually satisfying (and yes, perhaps even a bit kinky) moments together expand exponentially. I like to call this "building your own private sandbox." A custom-made playground just for you and those you choose to share it with, equipped with only the elements you enjoy playing with most and lacking anything that might feel unsafe or out of bounds. Now that you've gotten up close and personal with your own imagination, let's take a look at what dwells inside the minds (and sometimes on the screens) of others.

PornHub, Shakespeare, and Other Erotic Tales

Really thinking about what it is we enjoy sexually and what we think about when we daydream about sex can be a wonderful way to better get to know ourselves and our partners. While we live in a culture that is absolutely saturated with sexualized images and erotic content, we are not taught to think much about sex . . . and certainly not to talk about it. Sure, we know the mechanics of sexual intercourse, and, if we're lucky, some of us might even know what feels good to us, what induces arousal, turns us on, and gets us off. Research tells us that the majority of people, particularly women, do not. I think it's important to remind you here that *half* of women ages eighteen to thirty-five say that they have trouble reaching orgasm during partnered sex, and only 64 percent of women say that they had an orgasm during their last sexual encounter.[5]

2100 BCE

And Uchat . . . uncovered her nakedness, and let him enjoy her favors.

She was not ashamed, but yielded to his sensuous lust. She removed her garment, he lay in her arms,

And she satisfied his desire after the manner of women. He pressed his breast firmly upon hers.

For six days and seven nights, Enkidu enjoyed the love of Uchat.

—*The Epic of Gilgamesh*

Particularly for those in long-term relationships, we learn the shortcuts to pleasuring our partner: "If I move my hips like this, touch his chest like that, I know I can help him come." Sex becomes routine, even mechanical. Over time, we figure out our partner's climactic Konami Code and it becomes a standard rhythm: A-A-B-B-up-down-left-right-left-right-B-A-start and . . . blast off. It is quite possible that filling out the Fleshing Out Your Fantasies Worksheet might be the first time you have ever really sat and thought deeply about what it is that turns you on when you're all by yourself. Yet it has its own limitations because we do not know what we do not know. In some ways, this process is like going to a new restaurant featuring exotic cuisine we might never have tasted before. On the one hand, we might be able to make some general assumptions based on our overarching preferences. If I'm not a fan of squishy textures, I know not to order a custard, no matter what the flavor profile might be. On the other hand, if I know that I like the taste of chicken, how can I be so sure that I wouldn't also enjoy an entrée of pheasant or quail? One of the ways we try to inform our decision-making is by looking around the room and taking a peek at what other diners have on their plates. Which brings us to porn.

500s BCE

I slept, but my heart was awake. A sound! My beloved is knocking.

"Open to me, my sister, my love, my dove, my perfect one, for my head is wet with dew, my locks with the drops of the night."

I had put off my garment; how could I put it on? I had bathed my feet; how could I soil them?

My beloved put his hand to the latch, and my heart was thrilled within me.

I arose to my beloved, and my hands dripped with myrrh, my fingers with liquid myrrh, on the handles of the bolt.

I opened to my beloved . . .

—Song of Solomon 5:2–6a

Erotic images, ranging from pottery phalluses to obscene frescos, have existed in every culture around the world for as long as humanity has been creating art. While the ruins of Pompeii are most well known for the tragic castings of its fallen citizens, anthropologists are equally familiar with the city's public art, which depicted all manner of sexual creativity, variety, and expression. Monks would paint humorous yet explicit illustrations featuring autofellatio, bestiality, and all manner of fantastical erotica in the margins of the illuminated manuscripts they dedicated their lives to carefully writing out by hand. As soon as the printing press was invented, erotic tales of strict mistresses punishing naughty chambermaids proliferated. While most folks are familiar with the *Kama Sutra* and its depictions of tantric sexual positions, they are usually surprised to learn that Japan had a similar resource called shunga, or "pillow books," which contained erotic woodcuts depicting sexual images designed to inspire the reader to act out what they saw on the page. The Bible itself contains beautiful erotic poetry within the Song of Songs, along with some frankly obscene passages (Ezekiel 23:20) that have amused churchgoing adolescents for centuries.

2 CE

She who's known for her face, lie there face upwards. Let her back be seen, she whose back delights.

Milanion bore Atalanta's legs on his shoulders—if they're good-looking, that mode is acceptable.

Let the small be carried by a horse. Andromache, his Theban bride, was too tall to straddle Hector's horse.

Let a woman noted for her length of body, press the bed with her knees, arch her neck slightly.

She who has youthful thighs, and faultless breasts, the man might stand, she spread, with her body downwards.

—Ovid, *Ars Amorata*

Every innovation, from papyrus and clay to mailboxes and virtual reality headsets, have all pretty much instantly been used to create and disseminate erotica, which I believe shows us just how important this form of media can be for ourselves as humans. Something within us is deeply curious about what other people are doing in bed. This process of show-and-tell, in formats as public as a Hieronymus Bosch painting and as private as a Snapchat video clip, have been used to educate and amuse, titillate and inspire, for millennia. And the value of this exposure to the sexual lives of others has been predominantly recognized as a force for good. In the Babylonian Talmud, one of the sacred texts of the Jewish people, Tractate Berakhot 62a gives us an example of just this.

The Gemara relates that Rav Kahana entered and lay beneath Rav's bed. He heard Rav chatting and laughing with his wife, and seeing to his needs (i.e., having relations with her). Rav Kahana said, "The mouth of Rav is like one who has never eaten a cooked dish" (i.e., his behavior was lustful). Rav said to him, "Kahana, are you here? Leave!" Rav Kahana said to him, "But Rabbi, this too is Torah and I must learn."[6]

As a sex therapist, I love this story. The message—"This too is Torah [holy] and I must learn"—is a wonderfully impactful statement, especially for something written by religious scholars in 500 CE. In the same way that we can look around a restaurant and gain insight into what dishes seem appealing, we can leverage erotic content in order to start to fill in those gaps in our personal knowledge and experiences and create a mental map not only of what we already fantasize about but also of what new innovations we may be curious to explore. It is perhaps unsurprising that many of my clients are resistant to the idea that watching other people's sexual expression can be not only natural but beneficial. Particularly for those of us raised in North America, consuming erotic media is viewed as something to be done privately, if one must do it at all. We see news reports about various states declaring pornography a "public health crisis," and we hear worrisome anecdotes about revenge porn, human trafficking, and content containing images of minors. Though ethical erotica exists, these questions can feel complicated, perhaps even a bit scary. One can't be blamed for wanting to just avoid the whole thing entirely.

1350s CE

Isabetta was then set at liberty, and she and the Abbess returned to their beds, the latter with the priest and the former with her lover. She thenceforth arranged for him to visit her at frequent intervals, undeterred by the envy of those of her fellow nuns, without lovers, who consoled themselves in secret as best they could.

—Giovanni Boccaccio, *The Decameron*

In his book *His Porn, Her Pain*, Marty Klein, considered one of the world's foremost experts on pornography and the impact of erotica on relationships, identifies several key myths about viewing erotic materials. Among these are:

- Porn is mostly violent and misogynistic.

- Porn can cause erectile difficulties in men.

- Only men enjoy watching porn.

- Watching porn destroys otherwise happy, intimate relationships.

- Adult erotica is a "slippery slope" toward child sexual abuse material.

- Porn encourages violence against women.

- Porn somehow damages the brain or can even become addictive.[7]

When one dives into the research, as Klein does, we begin to see a complicated web of morality politics interwoven with public health policy. An entire industry of sex and pornography addiction treatment has risen up over the last few decades, one with a financial and, in many cases, spiritual stake in promoting the idea that erotica is dangerous, exploitative, and destructive. And yet "this too is Torah."

1594 CE

Petruchio: Who knows not where a wasp does wear his sting? In his tail.

Katharina: In his tongue.

Petruchio: Whose tongue?

Katharina: Yours, if you may talk of tails. And so, farewell.

Petruchio: What, with my tongue in your tail?

—William Shakespeare, *The Taming of the Shrew*,
Act 2, Scene 2

Many things that are known to be beneficial are prohibited by some faith traditions. The Church of Jesus Christ of Latter-Day Saints forbids the consumption of coffee by its members, even though the beverage is high in antioxidants and essential nutrients and has been shown to have many health benefits. Observant Jews do not consume any kind of shellfish, even though they represent one of our healthiest proteins, delivering omega-3 fatty acids with every bite. Christian Scientists refuse blood transfusions during surgeries, even when doing so might save their lives. It is only natural that one's personal faith and spiritual practice will inform their health and health-care choices; if your religious tradition is one that prohibits viewing erotic materials, I am not here to change your mind. Yet, in the same way that observant Jews do not advocate for laws that would ban the sale of lobster, we too must also recognize that something we personally choose not to consume may have benefits for those who do. So, what benefits have researchers found for those who enjoy erotic content?

1750 CE

By now I'm sure she's sucking at his delicious lips. Or already pounding his naked chest with her breasts.

Probably moaning like doves.

He's on top of her, and she's pressing against him. She's quite skilled to begin with. Maybe a bit shy,

But by now he's won her over, freed her

From any reticence. He's brought her close,

Touched her everywhere. Taught her everything.

—Muddupalani, *The Appeasement of Radhika*

Ten Benefits of Viewing Porn and Other Erotica

1. It relaxes and helps to lower cortisol (stress hormone) levels.[8]

2. It improves intimate communication in relationships and helps people set boundaries and ask for what they want.[9]

3. It offers exposure to (and can educate about) a variety of different styles, positions, and manners of sex.

4. It has been shown to increase libido and strengthen one's sexual desire.[10]

5. It exposes the viewer to a wide variety of body types, genders, races, and other diversities.[11]

6. It helps us figure out what we want, what turns us on, and what we might enjoy experiencing for ourselves.[12]

7. It shows the viewer that they are not alone; that no matter how niche their desire, there are others who enjoy the same thing(s) they do.

8. It can help us explore fantasies that might not be possible or that we might not want to act out in real life.[13]

9. It lets us see that the things we do in bed—our sounds and movements, our body fluids and reactions—are normal.

10. It allows traditionally marginalized folks, such as women, kinksters, people of color, and LGBTQIA+, to control the production of content portraying their bodies and their experiences.

1873–1876

Oh! How I must love you.

It is two o'clock in the morning. I have violated and well worked you, kissed, frigged, licked and sucked you, obliged you to yield to my desires—the most debauched, the most shamelessly degrading during the whole of the afternoon. All the afternoon, too, I have got you to suck my member and my testicles. I have made you pass your tongue between my toes and under my arms.

—William Lazenby, *The Romance of Lust*, Vol. 4

So what do you do if you're open to the idea that watching erotica either by yourself or together with your partner might have some benefits for you, but you're concerned about the ethics of watching porn? There are many ways to open the door to erotic entertainment without immediately jumping onto the internet and downloading the latest free-site videos. Here are a variety of strategies you can try, ranging from least to most explicit:

Start with mainstream novels that feature detailed scenes of love and lust. We've already talked about romance novels, but we don't have to stop there.

Helen Hardt and Cherise Sinclair both write relationship-focused love stories with BDSM themes. If you want steamy erotica without overtly BDSM elements, Zane's novels are for you. Helen Hoang writes amazing neurodivergent romance, while Katie Meyer specializes in sexy but not explicit "slow burn" modern love stories. Joanna Angel, herself a porn star, writes delightful choose-your-own-adventure–style sexy stories. George R. R. Martin's *Song of Fire and Ice* series and Diana Gabaldon's Outlander books both feature steamy sex set within beautifully written and highly literary worlds.

1954

But at the first word or sign from anyone you will drop whatever you are doing and ready yourself for what is really your one and only duty: to lend yourself. Your hands are not your own, nor are your breasts, nor, most especially, any of your bodily orifices, which we may explore or penetrate at will. You will remember at all times—or as constantly as possible—that you have lost all right to privacy or concealment, and as a reminder of this fact, in our presence you will never close your lips completely, or cross your legs, or press your knees together.

—Pauline Réage, *The Story of O*

Rosy app, a platform focused on women's sexual health, has a variety of erotic stories that you can sort by intensity/explicitness.

DIY storytelling lets you take control of the narrative. I often encourage my clients to write sexy short stories with themselves as the main character. This lets you control the degree of explicitness. One of my favorite couples activities is **pass-and-play storytelling**, where one person writes a sentence or two then passes it to their partner to add a sentence of their own. They continue to pass the story back and forth until they've created a collaborative story featuring elements of what turns them both on.

If the ideas and resources listed above seem too tame to you, if you aren't feeling creative, or if you're looking for stories that feature more specific scenarios, fetishes, or relationship dynamics, **Literotica.com** might be the place for you. Be cautious, though; this site aggregates user contributions, which means you can find stories about any theme you can possibly imagine . . . including some you might not want to. Finding a story online that highlights some of your favorite fantasy elements and then emailing it to your partner is safer than sending an unexpected naughty photo, but it can be just as exciting to receive. Alternatively, you could print a story and take turns reading it to each other in bed.

DipseaStories.com lets you sit back and enjoy listening to the story rather than having to play storyteller yourself. I encourage my clients to dim their lights, perhaps light some candles, then listen to a Dipsea tale while gently touching and massaging themselves and their partner. If you're more of a visual person, there are lots of women- and feminist-created erotica that can be enjoyed without worrying about the ethics of the production or the consent of those on screen. Among these ethical smut producers are **LustCinema**, **Bright Desire**, **FrolicMe**, and **Indie Porn Revolution**.

2021

. . . the man was breathing hard, worn out with wielding the whip and spanking her hard on the buttocks, whilst she felt herself filling up with strength and energy.

She had lost all shame now, and wasn't bothered about showing her pleasure; she started to moan, pleading with him to touch her, but, instead, the man grabbed her and threw her onto the bed.

—Paulo Coelho, *Eleven Minutes*

Regardless of whether you choose written, audio, or visual erotica, the key is to experience what it feels like to engage with this kind of content. You can do so alone, if it feels more comfortable, or with your partner. If you choose the latter, take turns picking out stories/scenes and have a conversation about what elements stood out to you and why it was chosen. Start with the questions below and then see where the discussion leads you. The key here is to approach each opportunity from a place of curiosity and encouragement, even if the scene shared ends up not being quite your "thing." It's also important to remember one of the BDSM community's favorite catch-phrases: "Your kink's not my kink, but your kink's okay."

Erotic Show-and-Tell Conversation Prompts

• What about this particular story/scene caught your eye when you found it?

• What did you like most about what we just read/watched? Is this something you'd like to try or just something you like to watch?

• What did you find yourself paying the most attention to when we watched/read this?

• Was there anything you saw that you didn't like? What was it that you found off-putting? Why?

• Have you ever had an experience similar to what we just watched/read? Would you be willing to tell me about that experience? (Feel free to modify this question if it makes you uncomfortable or jealous!)

BUILDING AN EROTIC VOCABULARY

Now that we've pinpointed our existing "fantasy road map" and have identified some detours from the norm that we might be curious about, it's time to continue building our erotic vocabulary. Erotic vocabulary refers to the words that we feel comfortable using when talking about sex, intimacy, sensation, and desire with our partners. For some of us, an erotic vocabulary is a natural part of how we speak, think, and communicate. If we were raised in homes where sexuality and the body were normal parts of the family conversation, we might have an expansive vocabulary of anatomical, sensory, and emotional words to draw upon. For those of us who were raised in households that considered sex taboo and the body an off-limits topic, our vocabulary might be much more limited. I have worked with a number of people who were raised to avoid using the correct anatomical terms for their body parts. As adults, they often feel uncomfortable, embarrassed, or even ashamed to discuss their bodies with me as their therapist, sometimes with their medical providers, and definitely with their partners. The negative emotions they experience when trying to discuss their bodies can lead to delayed medical intervention (such as when someone notices a lump in their testicle or experiences severe pain during menstruation), a lack of satisfaction in their relationships, and unnecessary guilt and shame. I have spent months with some clients helping them build and/or expand their erotic vocabularies before we can ever begin to address the challenges that brought them to my office in the first place.

Let's play a game right now and gauge the level of your own erotic vocabulary. Read the list of words below out loud. Then rate each one on a scale of 1 to 10, where 1 indicates an extreme discomfort saying the word and 10 represents total comfort. Underline the number that indicates how you feel when you *think* of the word. Circle the number that indicates how you feel about *saying* the word out loud. Consider sharing your results with your partner and asking them to complete the activity as well, then compare notes and see where your vocabularies overlap and where you each feel more or less comfortable. You can use these insights to tailor how you discuss sex and intimacy with each other moving forward. You can download and print this worksheet at stefanigoerlich.com/with-sprinkles-on-top -worksheets.html#/.

Erotic Vocabulary

Your Rating	Erotic Vocabulary Word	Your Partner's Rating
1 2 3 4 5 6 7 8 9 10	Breasts	1 2 3 4 5 6 7 8 9 10
1 2 3 4 5 6 7 8 9 10	Penis	1 2 3 4 5 6 7 8 9 10
1 2 3 4 5 6 7 8 9 10	Vulva	1 2 3 4 5 6 7 8 9 10
1 2 3 4 5 6 7 8 9 10	Vagina	1 2 3 4 5 6 7 8 9 10
1 2 3 4 5 6 7 8 9 10	Testicles	1 2 3 4 5 6 7 8 9 10
1 2 3 4 5 6 7 8 9 10	Scrotum	1 2 3 4 5 6 7 8 9 10
1 2 3 4 5 6 7 8 9 10	Princess	1 2 3 4 5 6 7 8 9 10
1 2 3 4 5 6 7 8 9 10	Anus	1 2 3 4 5 6 7 8 9 10
1 2 3 4 5 6 7 8 9 10	Clitoris	1 2 3 4 5 6 7 8 9 10
1 2 3 4 5 6 7 8 9 10	Nipples	1 2 3 4 5 6 7 8 9 10
1 2 3 4 5 6 7 8 9 10	Butt	1 2 3 4 5 6 7 8 9 10
1 2 3 4 5 6 7 8 9 10	Orgasm	1 2 3 4 5 6 7 8 9 10
1 2 3 4 5 6 7 8 9 10	Cock	1 2 3 4 5 6 7 8 9 10
1 2 3 4 5 6 7 8 9 10	Balls	1 2 3 4 5 6 7 8 9 10
1 2 3 4 5 6 7 8 9 10	Clit	1 2 3 4 5 6 7 8 9 10
1 2 3 4 5 6 7 8 9 10	Cum	1 2 3 4 5 6 7 8 9 10
1 2 3 4 5 6 7 8 9 10	Whore	1 2 3 4 5 6 7 8 9 10
1 2 3 4 5 6 7 8 9 10	Ass	1 2 3 4 5 6 7 8 9 10
1 2 3 4 5 6 7 8 9 10	Wet	1 2 3 4 5 6 7 8 9 10
1 2 3 4 5 6 7 8 9 10	Sex	1 2 3 4 5 6 7 8 9 10
1 2 3 4 5 6 7 8 9 10	Masturbation	1 2 3 4 5 6 7 8 9 10
1 2 3 4 5 6 7 8 9 10	Ma'am/Sir	1 2 3 4 5 6 7 8 9 10
1 2 3 4 5 6 7 8 9 10	Tease	1 2 3 4 5 6 7 8 9 10
1 2 3 4 5 6 7 8 9 10	Tingle	1 2 3 4 5 6 7 8 9 10
1 2 3 4 5 6 7 8 9 10	Throb	1 2 3 4 5 6 7 8 9 10
1 2 3 4 5 6 7 8 9 10	Ache	1 2 3 4 5 6 7 8 9 10
1 2 3 4 5 6 7 8 9 10	Naughty	1 2 3 4 5 6 7 8 9 10
1 2 3 4 5 6 7 8 9 10	Master/Mistress	1 2 3 4 5 6 7 8 9 10
1 2 3 4 5 6 7 8 9 10	Dick	1 2 3 4 5 6 7 8 9 10
1 2 3 4 5 6 7 8 9 10	Ride	1 2 3 4 5 6 7 8 9 10
1 2 3 4 5 6 7 8 9 10	Little Girl/Boy	1 2 3 4 5 6 7 8 9 10
1 2 3 4 5 6 7 8 9 10	Slut	1 2 3 4 5 6 7 8 9 10
1 2 3 4 5 6 7 8 9 10	Fuck	1 2 3 4 5 6 7 8 9 10
1 2 3 4 5 6 7 8 9 10	Cunt	1 2 3 4 5 6 7 8 9 10

It is likely that, for some of you, even reading many of these words felt uncomfortable. Talk to your partner about this as well. Ask each other:

- What words felt easiest for you to say? What words felt most difficult?

- How did you feel in your body when you were saying the difficult words out loud?

- What emotional reactions did you have while reading these words? Did any of them make you feel embarrassed? Ashamed? Aroused? Why or why not?

- Did reading these words bring up any memories for you? What images came to your mind while saying the words out loud?

- What kinds of words did your family use to describe sex and the body growing up? Do you feel like these choices affected how you think and/or talk about sex today?

SENSORY EXPLORATIONS

"Okay, great," I hear you thinking, "you've gotten me thinking about . . . and even saying . . . all kinds of sexual things. But this is all talk and no action. How on earth does this help me connect with my kinky partner?" Excellent point, dear reader! It's time to put our introspection into practice, so let's get physical! One of the classic exercises of sex therapy is called Sensate Focus Touch. It was originally developed by William Masters and Virginia Johnson, two pioneers of sexual health research. Originally practiced as part of an intensive two-week stay at their institute, the model was adapted by others over time to be practiced by partners at home, as homework assigned between sessions by their regular relationship therapist. The goal of Sensate Focus Touch was, and remains, counterintuitive. It's not an exercise in pleasure so much as of mindfulness. Heather Reznik, William Masters's last assistant before his retirement, describes it as an "exercise (that) is supposed to focus on non-demanding touching. There should be no expectations. Clients should only be focusing on sensation."[14]

In the spirit of Sensate Focus Touch and the practice of mindful body exploration without agenda or expectation, the next phase of exploration will involve giving and receiving various forms of sensation and touch. The exercises described below are inspired by Sensate Focus Touch and grounded in that same model of experience and communication, but they are not the traditionally structured model taught in formal sex therapy. Our goal here is more playful, creating the space for you and your partner to each explore various textures and pressures, erotic positions and tactile sensations. In practice, both of you will take turns giving and receiving sensation. The work of the person receiving that sensation is to engage mindfully with each sensory experience and to focus on how they respond (physically, mentally, and emotionally) to each. Then these thoughts and feelings are shared and discussed with the giving partner, who listens without judgment or critique. Then you switch roles and do it again. Let's break it down in more detail.

Playing with Textural Sensation

Gather four to six swatches of various tactile materials. These should ideally serve as a curated sensory experience inspired by your own fantasies as well as those of your partner. For example, if you've noticed that your daydreams tend to center around historical romance such as knight-and-princess themes, you might want to choose elements such as velvet and metal chain to create a sensation of opulence and armor. Perhaps your partner's fantasies run more along the lines of pirate king and captive wench, in which case you might want to choose materials such as cotton rope, leather, or even burlap with which to explore. If you aren't one for elaborate story lines in your fantasy life, feel free to choose materials from the list below and have your partner do the same. The only rationale you need to have for your selections is curiosity for that element.

Acupressure Needle Massager	Faux Fur	Natural Bristle Hairbrush
Aluminum Piping	Feathers/Feather Boa	Netting
Burlap	Flowers/Flower Petals	Painter's Tape
Corduroy	Jade Roller	Silk/Satin
Chainmail or Chain Links	Lace	Velvet
Cotton Rope/Braid	Latex/Rubber	Wire Scalp Massager
Denim	Leather	Wooden Paint Stir Stick

Once you have selected your materials, plan out a time when you and your partner can be uninterrupted for one hour. For the first fifteen minutes, you will lie undressed in a comfortable face-down position. Your partner will spend a few minutes stroking your body with each of the materials you selected together, making sure that you get to experience these textures across the whole of your body—from the soles of your feet to the top of your head. You may wish to experiment with lightly running each texture across your genitals. Because the delicate tissue of the labia and penis is sensitive, proceed with caution and avoid applying too much pressure or friction. If you chose six materials to play with, your partner should spend roughly two minutes with each. During this time, your job is simply to relax and focus on your own reactions to this experience. Take note of what feelings, both physical and emotional, come up for you:

- Are there textures that you have a strong negative reaction to?

- Are there sensations that you find surprisingly pleasurable?

- Did any of the textures bring up a memory for you?

- When your mind wanders during this process (and it will), what do you notice yourself thinking about?

After fifteen minutes, roll over to a comfortable position on your back and repeat the process, this time experiencing each sensation on your legs, belly, chest, and face. When you have had time to experience the chosen textures across the whole of your body (a process that should take roughly thirty minutes), it is time to switch and repeat the whole process for your partner. After you've spent this hour together giving and receiving sensation, take some time to relax and hold each other. Cuddle up and discuss what you noticed about this experience. Share the feelings that came up for you and talk about any textures you discovered that you might want to integrate into your nonfantasy intimate moments moving forward.

Playing with Pressure and Positioning Sensations

Once you've had time to play around with texture and explore the myriad ways in which your body can respond to varying materials, repeat the exercise but with a focus on temperature and pressure. I generally recommend that partners space this activity out a bit more, with one person receiving sensation one evening and the other taking their turn a day or two later. This portion of the exercise can occasionally bring up strong feelings for some participants (especially those with trauma histories), and it's important to give yourself and your partner the space and grace to go slowly, invoke their stop, and process their responses to these sensations. Repeat the exercise, slowly moving through each of the following positions. Hold them for one to two minutes, and give yourselves time to sit with the experience, both as giver and receiver.

1. The giving partner sits with their back against the bed or wall, arms and legs spread so that the receiving partner can sit between their legs. The giving partner wraps their arms and legs (if possible and desired) around the receiving partner and squeezes.

2. The receiving partner lies on the bed, curled up so that their legs and arms are beneath them. The giving partner then wraps their body atop the receiving partner, enfolding and enclosing them.

3. The receiving partner lies on the floor, face down in a comfortable position. The giving partner stands over them and gently places one foot on their back, across their shoulder blades. The giving partner should not put any body weight onto the receiving partner's back. Placement of their foot alone is sufficient. **Note:** For additional sensation, you can repeat this position with the giving partner's foot on the receiving partner's head—again, avoid placing pressure on the receiving partner.

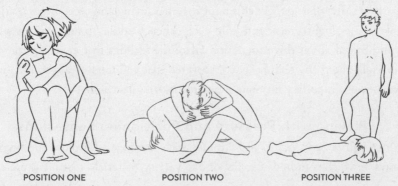

POSITION ONE   POSITION TWO   POSITION THREE

Artist: Natsu/Cry_Tm

110

4. The giving partner sits comfortably in a chair or on a sofa. The receiving partner sits comfortably at the giving partner's feet. The giving partner may choose to stroke the receiving partner's hair.

5. The receiving partner kneels on all fours (hands and knees) while the giving partner strokes their hair and back. **Note:** For added sensation, the giving partner could sit and place their feet on the receiving partner's tabled back.

6. The receiving partner lies on their back in a comfortable position on the bed while the giving partner straddles their hips, placing one knee on either side of the receiving partner's body. The giving partner holds both of the receiving partner's wrists above their head, exerting light pressure.

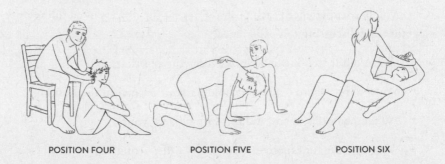

POSITION FOUR   POSITION FIVE   POSITION SIX

Artist: Natsu/Cry_Tm

7. The receiving partner sits comfortably on the bed or floor. The giving partner gathers a bedsheet in their hands and wraps it around the receiving partner, exerting gentle pressure to create a squeezing sensation.

8. The giving partner sits comfortably on a chair or sofa while the receiving partner sits in their lap. The giving partner wraps their arms around the receiving partner and holds them gently.

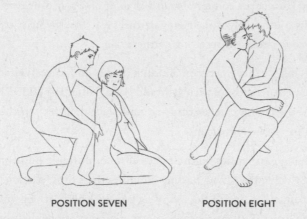

POSITION SEVEN   POSITION EIGHT

Artist: Natsu/Cry_Tm

Once you have experienced each position, repeat the process of cuddling up together and discussing this experience:

- What did it feel like to be in the receiving position?

- How did it feel to be the one holding your partner in the position?

- What memories, if any, did this bring up for you?

- Was anything unexpectedly enjoyable? Off-putting?

- Did you need to invoke your stop? Can you express why?

- Did you discover positions you may wish to try again?

I suggest that you do each of these activities several times to give you opportunities to notice changes in your responses. Some touches or textures might feel lovely early in one's menstrual cycle (for example) while being off-putting later on in the month. Our reactions might vary depending upon time of day or state of health. Exploring each of these fully gives you and your partner lots of information that you can use for the next stage of our *Sprinkles* discovery.

Negotiating Desire

Shelley: I've been interested in being dominated since I was about twenty years old. I love the idea of bondage, but it becomes difficult with my physical disability. I've never been able to fully relax into a comfortable position for bondage. I started focusing on my senses for play. I like to have my sight removed (eyes closed, blindfolded, or pillow over face) because it allows me to focus on my physical sensations.

Brad: My kink, hypnokink, where I am the subject on the receiving end of consensual nonconsent/brainwashing me, does not lend itself to being aggressive. I'm not the aggressor in sexual situations.

Shelley: I'm 100 percent aware of his boundaries and my boundaries during play. I tend to hyperfocus on my boundaries and stop at the slightest bit of anxiety or frustration.

Brad: We didn't start off in a kinky relationship. Our sexual relationship evolved over time in discussing our desires and fantasies. It brings value in that we are more connected with each other. Our communication has deepened overall. The drawback is that we both are mainly submissives.

Shelley: I would love to feel more comfortable with embracing my sexuality overall. I grew up with shame around sexuality, so I have this background noise of disapproval from others.

Brad: Communication is key. Bringing up what you like little by little depending on what you like. Most partners are interested in trying things. Incorporating what they like into your kink is a great way to keep both partners involved.

Shelley: Don't shame your partner. It can be overwhelming exploring kink with your partner if you're not kinky. Your partner's desires may be off-putting at first, but I challenge you to question why they're off-putting. Is it shame around sexuality?

Is it that it isn't the "norm" for others/society? Listen to what your partner shares and then ask to process it on your own before responding. Ask questions about their kink as well. You'll learn more and it'll help you two to explore sexuality together.

Brad: Be open and willing. Sometimes the things your partner likes may sound weird at first but can be fun once you begin exploring. If you don't like it at any point, communicate and set your boundaries. It's better to explore than to reject your partner's kink.

MORE TO READ ON THIS TOPIC

Ethical Porn for Dicks: A Man's Guide to Responsible Viewing Pleasure

David J. Ley, PhD

God Loves Sex: An Honest Conversation about Sexual Desire and Holiness

Dan B. Allender and Tremper Longman III

His Porn, Her Pain: Confronting America's PornPanic with Honest Talk about Sex

Marty Klein, PhD

5

Taste-Testing Other Flavors

I hope that you've enjoyed working (alone and together) to figure out what you already like—those scenarios, sensations, and ideas that are already part of our internal erotic recipe whether we think about them consciously or not. There is tremendous value in understanding ourselves physically, emotionally, and relationally. We see that reflected in BDSM negotiations, where partners take a few minutes to define their likes and limits before entering into an intimate moment together. Here, we're going to introduce the idea of experimenting with some other ideas (perhaps those introduced by your kinky partner) in ways that feel safe and comfortable for you. One of my favorite quirks of the BDSM community is its use of the word *play* to describe intimate experiences. I want to lean in to the idea of playfulness and playing together as a way to learn and grow as partners and sexual beings. The idea of sex as play is not as common as I would like it to be within the "vanilla" world. Too often we are socialized to look at sex as an obligation to fulfill, a luxury to aspire to have, or simply a biological urge to be endured. Before we start to think about reframing intimacy as an opportunity for playfulness, we need to consider what gets in the way of this mindset: the mental and emotional baggage that we carry with us into our conversations about desire.

ASKING FOR WHAT WE WANT

Most of us are not good at asking for what we want. Many women are socialized to be deferential and modest, both as household and intimate partners. We are taught that we should be "polite," which often is interpreted to mean undemanding. Meanwhile, many men are socialized to take on the role of leader and seducer. "A real man" should never need to explicitly state what he needs; he should take it. Or his partner should be attuned enough to his masculine leadership that they know intuitively how to provide it. This still rather patriarchal socialization fails to account for the spectrum of male and female (and other) identities and personalities. Likewise, it fails to offer a path forward for those of us who have unmet needs or unspoken desires. Some of us are taught to ignore our own wants while prioritizing the desires of others. Others are told that they should simply *claim* what they want and that everyone will swoon. Meanwhile, a sizable portion of the population is excluded from the narrative entirely, simply because they don't fall into a heteronormative box. At the end of the day, many of us are left floundering, ill-equipped to speak to the hole of longing we experience and unsure of how our partner would respond, even if we could.

Unmet needs or unspoken desires can quickly be transformed into conflicts when we don't have tools to address them. The empty space, that secret want, and the urgent calling within us can start to fester into resentment and animosity—unless we find a way to share it with our partner. In other words, the stakes here can become very high very quickly. The emotional narrative we create for ourselves when we do not have the words to express our desires to our partner is shaped by layers of history and experience that may or may not be directly tied to our unspoken longing. Often there is a nuance to what we crave that we don't feel like we have the right words to explain. It all feels like *just so much* and our voices fail us.

Let's spend a few moments dialing down the intensity of these conversations by drawing inspiration from something most folks are far more comfortable expressing: their food preferences. This might feel slightly ridiculous on the surface, but the sexual appetite and our cravings for food are not dissimilar. C. S. Lewis once used the analogy of a slowly revealed hamburger to critique the idea of sexualized entertainments like strip clubs.[1] His point was that our desire for sex was no different than our desire for food and should be treated just as matter-of-factly, neither eroticized nor denied. And he believed that turning the naked body into something provocative or titillating made about as much sense as whooping and hollering as a napkin was pulled away to reveal a juicy burger. After all, in his mind sex and hunger were simple, basic bodily urges. If Lewis were alive today, he might face-palm the first time he saw the Food

Network, an entire channel devoted to the art of the culinary tease! I might disagree with his stance on the erotic, but I find his hamburger analogy to be quite useful to our purposes here. What would it look like if we unpeeled the layers of influence that affect our abilities to speak our desire, using Lewis's hamburger as our guide?

Exploring Our Influences

OUR UNMET NEEDS: Beneath every fantasy lies a need that we believe the experience will fulfill for us. Later on in this chapter, you'll find a list of needs that people seek out intimacy in order to fulfill. Some of these will resonate with you. Others might seem quite different from your own experiences with intimacy, and for many of us the need might be even more specific, even more personal. Understanding what we truly desire is key to asking our partner for what we want.

> *What is it about a hamburger that feels exactly right for me right now? Why do I want this and not a steak? Or a hot dog? What craving will the hamburger—specifically the hamburger—fill for me.*

OUR EMOTIONAL REACTIONS: We understand the idea of sexual frustration—the irritation/rejection combo pack that can occur when we are aroused and our partner simply isn't feeling it. Recognizing the emotional reactions that our unspoken desires are bringing up for us can be key to speaking these needs to our partner in a way that feels sexy and inviting rather than conjuring anger or hurt. If we begin to notice that our unmet needs and unspoken desires are connected to feelings of sadness, upset, or hurt? It becomes all the more important to find a way to ask our partner for what we want before this resentment undermines the relationship entirely.

> *How do I feel when I'm hungry? Not the physical sensations of growling stomachs and low blood sugar but the emotional cues I barely notice unless I'm really paying attention. Does hunger make me angry? Does the act of eating evoke a sense of safety that comes from understanding what it means to not know where my next meal will come from?*

OUR SELF-PERCEPTION AND SELF-ESTEEM: Our self-perception is how we assume others view us. Our self-esteem is how we feel about ourselves. Often used interchangeably, these are fluid concepts that can and do influence each other but represent two distinct perspectives. If we see ourselves as unworthy, unattractive, awkward, or prudish, this is going to influence how we assume others perceive us as well. And if we leave our encounters with the other people in our lives feeling as if our presence is valued, that we contribute something positive in our professional life and make an impact in the lives of others, we will move through the world and interact with others accordingly. Our internal understanding of who we are and how others see us directly affects how we experience our own desires and confidence in sharing them with others.

In some families, women serve their spouses the best cut of meat before eating themselves. In some families, the children might eat a simpler meal (hot dogs or hamburgers) rather than the more grown-up fare, like steak, consumed by their parents. Do I feel like I deserve to eat the best food on the table or have I been told to be content with what's leftover when the important people have been served? Do I feel worthy of sitting down to an elegant meal or should I just eat a plain hamburger patty standing alone over the kitchen sink? Do I feel like I'm allowed to want what I want?

OUR UNSPOKEN EXPECTATIONS: Often tied directly to our culture and socialization, unspoken expectations are those rules and behaviors that we assume are universal. These can be as simple as door-holding protocols between men and women entering a building and as complicated as the way we date, give and receive love, initiate sex, and maintain relationships with our partners. Most of us assume that we don't need to speak our unspoken expectations because the other people around us should simply *know* that this is how a reasonable, kind, and healthy person should behave. We often carry our unspoken expectations with us from our families of origin into our adult relationships, which can pose problems since our partners typically come from different family cultures and bring their own "universal" truths with them as well. These can be the root source of many conflicts around sex and intimacy because they seem like things we shouldn't have to say to our partner. I tell the couples I work with that when it comes to unspoken expectations, we have two options: speak them or stop expecting them. Either option is a valid choice, but eventually we have to choose.

In some families, the grill represents the man's domain. Mom might cook dinner 340 nights a year, but during the summer months, Dad's in charge—the Hamburger King, as it says there on his apron. What would my partner say if I mentioned that I grew up with my dad using a charcoal grill and so his preferred high-end propane device really doesn't give me the flavor I want? How would they react if I told them that I think hamburger meat is revolting and I'd really kill for a veggie patty? Do I feel capable of telling them that the hamburgers they prepare, while perfect to their taste, are overseasoned? Isn't a hamburger just a hamburger? Is it even worth mentioning . . . even though I walk away hungry on these grilled-dinner nights?

OUR PAST EXPERIENCES: Studies have shown that over the course of our lives, the average person will have approximately seven to eight relationships and seven to ten sexual partners. On average, two of these relationships will last more than a year. We will have four dates that qualify as "disasters" and at least two heartbreaks. Most of us will be cheated on once and will likely cheat once ourselves.[2] In other words, we bring *a lot* of experience to our present relationships—and not all of it is pleasant. When we are holding an unmet need or unspoken desire, it is important to consider how our feelings are being influenced by these past experiences. Are we used to having our feelings minimized and our needs ignored? If so, we might be less likely to trust our current partner to respond positively. Have we stretched our comfort zone for a partner in the past, only to have them blow right past our boundaries and take a mile instead of the offered inch? This might make us less open to meeting our partner's needs in the current relationship. It's not wrong to rely on past experiences in order to inform our decision-making processes; that's the definition of how learning occurs. But being mindful of how and when our past experiences are creating barriers to trust and engagement with our current partner can be an important part of not only expressing our needs to them but also being willing and able to hear them share their desires with us.

Nearly every hamburger I've eaten in my life has been delicious. In fact, they were my favorite food growing up! Until that time in college when I ate a burger that was just a little too rare . . . and ended up with a wicked case of food poisoning. It was so bad that I had to miss my exams and go to urgent care for a fluid IV. No matter how delectable a hamburger has looked since then, I just can't bring myself to eat one. The mere look of them brings up waves of nausea that I can't ignore. I know my spouse doesn't get it. In their mind, they're a quick, affordable way to feed the kids and me after a long day of work. But I start to feel anxious and wary just smelling them when I walk in the door.

OUR UNRESOLVED ISSUES: For many of us, our past experiences leave us with scars that we carry with us into the present moment. These might be childhood abuse or neglect, sexual or relational traumas, relationships of all kinds that ended without closure or kindness, and many other experiences that influence how we move through the world and engage with others today. None of these feelings are wrong, and many make perfect sense in the context of our experiences. Our task is to understand our histories and the way that we carry these stories and experiences within us—to be aware of how we react when situations arise that remind us of something difficult from our past, and to be willing to seek out the personal support necessary to parse out present challenges from past experiences so that we are able to be connected and engaged in our bodies and relationships today.

When I was a child, I loved chicken nuggets more than any other food. The little dino shapes made me happy and always felt like a special treat. On the nights when my parents served hamburgers, it felt like a crushing disappointment. First of all, burgers never looked like brontosauruses, no matter how hard my imagination worked. Second, the texture was weird, and I didn't like it. But my parents had a "clean-plate rule" and would not let us leave the table until we'd eaten everything we'd been served. I can't count how many nights I fell asleep at the table, stubbornly refusing to eat that hamburger. My parents never gave in. They'd let me sit there all night, then serve me the cold meat again for breakfast. I'm sure it's weird that a healthy, red-blooded American doesn't like hamburgers. And it's really not about the taste anymore. It's the memory . . . eating a hamburger as an adult feels like giving in when I'm finally old enough to set my own rules and say NO—I don't want the damn thing and I'm not going to eat it!

OUR PRIVATE BIASES: We all have biases. Some are fairly benign ("I don't find T-shirts and shorts attractive; I prefer partners who like to dress up"), while others are more insidious ("People like that are disgusting"). Recognizing where we might be categorizing people or behaviors in ways that are stigmatizing or hostile ("A gentleman would never do such a thing" or "Anyone who likes that activity is a pervert") is an important part of our ability to be fully present and supportive for our partners and our own well-being. Being able to accept ourselves completely, including our wants and desires, is crucial to overcoming the shame and embarrassment that we might feel when we consider asking our partner for what we want. It's always okay to have turnoffs. It's when we fall into patterns of categorizing people or behaviors as good or bad in and of themselves that we run the risk of perpetuating harm against others simply because their *thing* (whatever it might be) isn't one we share.

Growing up, my parents were big into the outdoors, and we grilled most nights from April until October. One year when I was about nine, our class went on a field trip to a farm and I got to bottle-feed a baby cow. Some of the other kids started jokingly calling it "Baby Burger." That was the first time it clicked for me that my favorite food came from this sweet little animal currently eating out of my hand. When I got home that night, I told my parents that meat was disgusting and that I would never eat another baby burger again. Thirty years later, I've kept my word. I know hamburgers taste delicious but, morally and ethically, I will not touch them.

BRINGING BACK PLAYTIME

You'll notice that most of the factors that influence our appetites occur well before an age when we understand what desire truly is. Our feelings are shaped by variables such as family relationships, cultural practices, significant experiences, or key memories that might be only tangentially related to the subject at hand. As with food preferences, the messages both overt and subtle that we receive about sex influence our understanding of what intimacy "should" be before we're ever old enough to form a conscious opinion about our own sexual desires.

For my clients, one of the biggest mental barriers to bringing playfulness back to intimacy is the fact that most of them were never taught that sex should be playful at all. Most of us receive a sex education that offers a very clinical, rather linear framework for what sex should look like, and it goes something like this:

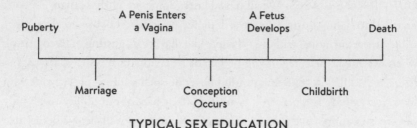

TYPICAL SEX EDUCATION

If we're lucky enough to attend a school that offers "comprehensive" sex education, which adds a bit of hyperbole and risk mitigation to the mix, our mental model for human sexuality might look more like this:

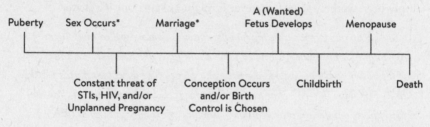

*Gender of partners unspecified

BETTER SEX EDUCATION

Both of these frameworks do a disservice to young people and leave adults wholly unprepared for the reality of what it means to be a sexual being. Both of them still assume one of two goals for "successful" sex: ejaculation for him and conception for her. Rarely is the topic of orgasm discussed at all. And while schools and teachers will acknowledge that not all students want to have children, the lessons still focus on the biology of reproduction rather than the psychology of healthy intimate relationships. And most people *will* have multiple intimate relationships! We rarely have only one marriage these days, much less only one significant partner. The vast majority of us date casually, sometimes have sex with people we have no desire to be with long term, and often have sex with no one but ourselves and starting at a younger age than many people realize. In fact, for most people, the reality looks much more like this:

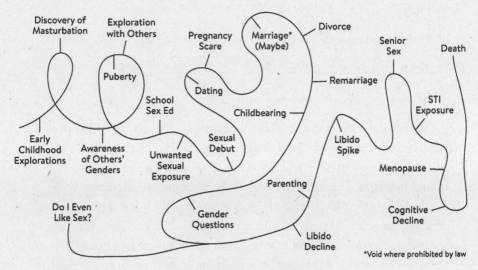

ACTUAL SEX EXPERIENCES

In other words, sex and relationships are much more complicated than most of us are taught to believe. Even as we live out the milestones of experiences such as making out in middle school or marrying after college, wondering if we like girls (or if we might not be a girl), or catching our toddler playing with their genitals . . . we still assume that we are meant to be following that linear path outlined for us in grade school. Any deviation from this procreative road map feels strange, confusing, or even sinful. But the simple fact is that for most of our lives, sex is not about the reproductive cycle. *It's about connectivity, intimacy, and fun.*

Collaborative Communication

So how do we bring play back into our sex lives? Or how do we start to add playfulness into a space where it has never been considered? This is where we put all of the insights and knowledge you've gained over the course of this chapter into practice. And it starts with how we communicate with our partners. Collaborative communication (also called nonviolent communication) was developed by the psychologist Marshall Rosenberg in the 1960s and '70s. He taught his clients a simple method for speaking up about difficult topics using principles of person-centered therapy. This method includes four key pieces:

Observation

Feeling (or Impact)

Need

Request

The Observation is simply that—a statement that tells the other person what behavior you've observed. I like to tell my clients that there are "no adjectives or expletives" in collaborative communication, so the observation should ideally be a neutral statement about what has occurred.

The Feeling piece lets you tell the other person how the behavior you observed affected you. It lets you tell them the way their behavior made you feel. This is a short, declarative statement that lets them ask clarifying questions ("I don't get why that would bother you so much") but doesn't open up the door to debate around your experience ("You don't feel hurt right now").

The Need is often the hardest part for folks to pin down. We want to tell them what we want from them ("I need you to not do that again"), when really the need is focused not on them but on us. This requires the speaker to really consider what they need most in this moment, and those needs can often be abstract or intangible. "I need to know you respect me" or "I need to feel safe," for example. The need is usually not something the other person can physically give to you. Your partner cannot, for example, run to the store and pick you up a can of safety to meet your needs. That's where the request comes in.

The Request is your opportunity to provide a suggestion for how they can best meet your needs at this moment. So, if you need to feel safe (to stick with our example), you might tell them, "I need you to ask me before you touch me." The trick here is the fact that *no* is always a valid answer. I teach my clients that *no* is sacred. We respect the no's we get from others because we want our own no's to be respected as well. But a no does not end this conversation! Rather, it serves as a lead-off point, because you still feel the way you feel and need what you need. Now you can have a conversation about how best to meet that need—even if it's not in the way you'd originally requested.

What does this look like in practice? Let's use a common complaint I hear in my work with clients: unwanted touching. I might help a husband tell his wife:

"When you tickle me while I'm trying to do the dishes, it makes me feel incredibly nervous. I need to feel safe while handling our knives and breakables. Could you please not tickle me in the kitchen?"

She may respond by telling him that she never realized that she was making him nervous when she tickled him and agree immediately to stop. She might also come back and ask:

"Well, what if you're in the kitchen but not doing dishes. Can I tickle you then?"

This allows her to seek clarification around the feeling and the need, and they are then able to work together to negotiate a way to meet that need that works for both of them. Because there are no adjectives or expletives involved in the process, it is easier for both the speaker and the listener to set aside hostility and defensiveness and to work together to address the concern.

I love collaborative communication and have taught it to everyone from young children and their parents to corporate executives. The format is the same no matter who you are, and while it can feel a little stilted or formal at first, once it becomes a part of your communication habit, it is easy to fall into naturally when difficult moments arise. Some of our most difficult conversations happen around sexuality and intimacy, and this gives us a tool to address our needs and boundaries with our partners in a way that is free of hostility and judgment.

"When I find you watching porn featuring rough sex, it makes me feel scared. I need to know that you will respect my limits, even around stuff that I know you enjoy. Can you please reassure me that you won't be rough with me in real life?"

Collaborative communication is a wonderful way to not only talk about what has gone wrong but also to highlight what went well. For example:

"When you called me your princess in bed the other night? It made me feel cherished and small in a way I really loved. I need to know that you will protect me, even when vulnerable and exposed. Can you please use that term, and others like it, outside of the bedroom too?"

Once we are able to recognize that sex fills a wide variety of needs beyond the simply procreative purpose we are taught in school, we can use collaborative communication to broaden the way we talk about sex and intimacy with our partner. We might tell them that we want to have sex or engage in some specific sexy thing because we need . . .

- to feel loved
- reassurance
- comfort
- connection
- stress relief
- exercise
- physical touch
- a self-esteem boost
- to express gratitude
- to celebrate
- to try something new
- to alleviate depression
- to feel powerful

- to feel protected
- spiritual transcendence
- to conceive
- money/gifts
- pain relief
- to clear our mind
- an orgasm
- to keep our partner from straying
- romance
- adventure
- risk/danger
- bonding

Once we've gotten into the habit of using collaborative communication with folks outside of the bedroom, we can use this same format to weave in elements of our fantasy and sensation explorations in order to ask our partner for what we desire in a way that is clear, direct, and unashamed. This might come easily to you as you begin to build your collaborative communication muscles, or you might still struggle to verbalize your desires to your partner simply because of the deeply intimate nature of these conversations. That's okay! Talking about sex is a skill we build over time.

One of the strengths of the BDSM community is their ability to be comfortable talking about sex: what they want, what they don't want, and how to accomplish both. The process of negotiating a scene starts with an acknowledgment that isn't made in those eighth-grade biology classes: that sex can be fun without being goal-oriented and that pleasure can occur without penetration, much less orgasm. In fact, most kinky people engage in careful conversations before playing with one another that (rather serendipitously) align nicely with the collaborative communication model. Indeed, many negotiation conversations use a structured framework (like a checklist) that lets each person fill in the blanks to state their desires and expectations for a scene. These are discussed, explained, clarified, negotiated, and then respected—very much like the process of collaborative communication. These conversations might include things like:

"When we have sex, I need to know that you are completely focused on me."

"My focus tonight is on having an orgasm."

"I want to feel desired and adored, and one of the best ways to get me there is to stroke my hair, to say things like 'How can I please you?' to me while you massage my feet."

"I love the feeling of being elaborately dressed up and would love to include that in our play together."

"When you gently trace my body with your fingertips, it makes me feel like you worship me, and I really want that to be a part of our time together."

"On the other hand, I don't want you to hold my wrists because it makes me feel out of control and that's not what I want this time."

"I want you to know that when I watch you lick me, I get really tingly and wet and that is one of my favorite parts of being with you."

"I love seeing your mouth fall open when we touch each other, and I really love your fingers in my hair."

"Sometimes I like to imagine that I am an ancient Greek deity and you are my priest, and I think it would be really hot if we could play around more with that idea together."

"When you call me Goddess, it feeds that fantasy for me and my body gets flush and warm."

"I think it would be fun if you fed grapes to me on the back porch while the sun sets before we play."

"I really want you to be gentle and worship me. And afterward, I want to relax in a bubble bath while you wash my hair."

One critique of collaborative communication that I've heard over the years is that it can feel a little bit like Mad Libs to new users—a standard script you read with a few blanks to fill in along the way. I loved Mad Libs growing up and think that this is more of an apt description than an actual criticism. At their best, Mad Libs gave us a simple tool that brought us closer to the people with us. They let us relax and know that we're not expected to create storytelling gold out of whole cloth. They let us create a mutually enjoyable experience simply by filling in the blanks. To that end, I'm including a Mad Lib of my own at the end of this chapter. Based on our earlier example, it will let you weave all of the elements that you've explored over the course of the last exercises into one descriptive and detailed fantasy proposal that you can share with your partner. But before we get there, let's look at some other strategies for bringing playfulness, creativity, and perhaps even a little bit of kink into your relationship.

KINK AS PLAYTIME

Often when we think of BDSM, our thoughts turn immediately toward preconceived notions of violence, aggression, degradation, or even danger. We assume that kink means suffering (physically and/or emotionally) for our partner's pleasure. It's often a pleasant surprise for many of my clients, when they first begin to explore the world of BDSM, to discover the joy, laughter, even silliness that exists in so many kinky spaces. While researching my last book, *Kink-Affirming Practice: Culturally Competent Therapy from the Leather Chair*, I interviewed over two hundred kinky people and asked them to describe their relationship dynamic in two to three words. The interviewees represented a cross section of the BDSM world—brats and tamers, dominants and submissives, caregivers and their pets or littles, folks who live in regimented 24/7 master/slave hierarchies, as well as sadists and masochists who prioritize sensation over power exchange—and all chose surprisingly consistent words to describe dramatically different relationship dynamics. The top five descriptors that kinky people used to describe their relationships were *love*, *care*, *playful*, *fun*, and *safe*.[3]

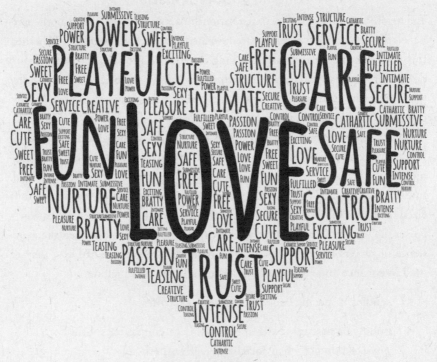

BDSM WORD MAP

Many of the vanilla partners I see in my practice express both relief and genuine delight when they begin to explore the ways in which BDSM play can become a positive force in their relationships, and not just erotically but outside of the bedroom as well. Why might this be so?

In his book *The Erotic Mind*, Jack Morin identifies what he describes as the four cornerstones of eroticism: longing and anticipation, violating prohibitions, searching for power, and overcoming ambivalence.[4] Perhaps unsurprisingly, many aspects of BDSM play fall into one or more of these four categories. As a result, partners who experiment with integrating elements of kink (which may or may not involve activities some might consider painful or upsetting) into their sexual or relational lives often report experiencing not only greater sexual satisfaction but also a closer relationship bond.[5] What do Morin's cornerstones look like in practice within a kinky relationship dynamic?

Longing and Anticipation

The healthiest and frankly sexiest relationships are those in which both partners look forward with eagerness to the time when they are reunited. Whether this occurs at the airport during a long-distance relationship or at the front door after a busy workday, intimacy thrives when we crave each other. We are wired for relationships. Beginning as newborns, we are entirely reliant on our caregivers for food and comfort, safety and love. So dependent are we on the responsiveness of others that our brains learn to crave their attention and to predict the circumstances under which that desire will be fulfilled. This cognitive cycle of need—Morin writes that "longing always directs its attention towards what's missing or in short supply"—and prediction becomes eroticized through a lifetime of sensory experiences into longing and anticipation.[6] Power play and power exchange leverage these emotions to heighten the experience of players within a kink scene. Some examples of how BDSM play is used to enhance and reinforce longing and anticipation include:

- sending a specific daily photo to your partner

- finding opportunities for meaningful eye contact or subtle physical contact when socializing with others

- homecoming rituals (such as kneeling at the door awaiting the dominant's return) that foster a sense of anticipation and connection

- varying sensations (such as interspersing surprise pinches in with gentle strokes of the body) during foreplay and sex

- teasing, edging, and orgasm denial during sex

Violating Prohibitions

This is what Morin describes as "the naughtiness factor"—that thrill we get when we do something a little transgressive. When we do something that's perceived as "bad," our body responds in a way very similar to how we react to danger—in this case, the "danger" of getting caught. Our awareness of risk activates the parasympathetic nervous system, which reacts just as it would if we were lost on the savannah, scanning the horizon for predatory lions. Our senses narrow and become heightened, our brain flips into hypervigilance, scanning the scene for any risk, and our body experiences that rush of adrenaline that sends tingles throughout our limbs. Because of these innate biological reactions, crossing some boundaries and engaging in play that carries the perception of danger without the actual threat can enhance the experience of sex and intimacy emotionally ("We're in this together! Don't get caught!") and physiologically. Our brain can't differentiate between real and make-believe lions. Creating situations that allow us to experience that novel thrill without genuine risk can be great fun for the thrill seekers among us.

The prohibitions we violate can take many forms. Exhibitionism and voyeurism are popular forms of transgressive play. For some, this takes the form of watching an online performer's livestream or even engaging in anonymous interactive exhibitionism through sites that consensually connect folks who want to be seen with those who want to watch. Visiting clubs where guests can watch others engage in sexual activity or allow others to watch them can scratch that itch in a way that maintains the consent of everyone involved. Others might use role-play to experiment with taboos—those rules that society or our culture tells us are sacrosanct, especially those around expected social roles and boundaries. The stepbrother/stepsister dynamic in so many erotic videos leans in to the illusion of violating incest taboos, for example, while offering the plausible deniability of "step" that works to counterbalance our aversion to violating this particular culture norm. The naughty schoolgirl and strict principal or lapsed clergyperson and seductive demoness are popular Halloween costumes because they lean in to this idea of subverting role prohibitions. These tropes can feel uncomfortable or off-putting for some folks because they play with "problematic" power dynamics. For others, that discomfort is a part of the appeal. Another way we can stimulate our parasympathetic nervous system and play with prohibitions is by racing the clock. When we role-play a scene in which we must finish the act quickly or risk getting caught (like horny teenagers rushing to finish before their parents get home from work), we create a fantasy that fosters excitement and the thrill of someone catching us being "bad." Sex in the office supply closet during the company holiday party or in the car at Lover's Lane, hoping the cops don't show up, are scenarios that feed this particular transgressive thrill. Some ways that you can add elements of violating prohibitions into your relationship include:

- Pick a position, phrase, toy, or wardrobe item that feels "bad" or "naughty" to you and try using it the next time you're being intimate with yourself or with your partner. See how it makes you feel to break a rule.

- Find an erotic story that features characters violating a prohibition you find sexy but that you might not be comfortable acting on. Take turns reading aloud to each other.

- Text your partner a few minutes into their commute home and let them know you'll be masturbating in the bedroom. See if they can "catch" you before you finish.

- Make a date to have sex in a spot you would not usually consider. On the kitchen table, a few hours before family dinner? In a by-the-hour motel? Up against the window with the bedroom lights off?

- Visit a strip club or peep show together and buy your partner a lap dance.

Searching for Power

You might have noticed a theme throughout this book—the idea of power exchange. And sure, this is the most obvious way that we can interpret Morin's third cornerstone. On a subtler level, we can begin to think about the diverse ways in which power is sought after and expressed in our society through high-power jobs, high-powered cars, fame, affluence, beauty, and authority, to name just a few. Morin observes that even the most vanilla people talk about sex in terms of power: being on top or being on bottom; feelings of safety or helplessness and how the sense of our own power in a given scene or moment informs our erotic expression. For many vanilla partners of kinky people, not being able to understand our partner's needs or relate to their desires can cause a sense of disconnection that might leave us feeling powerless or out of control. We feel helpless, out of our depth, and these feelings can feel threatening to our relationship and our sense of self. Moving toward a more intentional search for power—through communication, curiosity, experimentation, and play—can create a space where we can explore what power means for our partner and reclaim it for ourselves. This might look like:

- Being mindful of the types of power we encounter in our daily lives and noticing the forms power can take and the ways we engage with them.

- Paying attention to where we have power, both *over* and *with* others, and how we feel about this. (*Power over* might include leadership roles at work or within social organizations. *Power with* might include coparenting decisions or an employee-owned business.)

- Noticing the types of television or movie characters that turn us on or arouse our interest. Observing the qualities they have in common as well as the reactions we have to them.

- Talking to our partner about the way that power is shared within the relationship. Who is responsible for what within the household and, more importantly, why?

- Claiming power in the bedroom—making a conscious effort to ask our partner for what we want, to move in ways that feel good for us, to own our right to pleasure.

Overcoming Ambivalence

When I first introduce the concept of overcoming ambivalence to the couples that I work with, I often see the more vanilla partner become wary. Upon first listen, it sounds like I'm about to suggest a process by which their partner and I cajole them into moving past their boundaries and into a space where they feel pressured to acquiesce to a kinky request, even if their heart isn't in it. Good news! That is not what Morin had in mind when he laid out this cornerstone. Overcoming ambivalence is not "I really *really* don't like this idea but giving in would make them so happy . . . I should just do it." (On a related note, coercion of any kind should never happen during your counseling process!) Rather, the key element of overcoming ambivalence is that delicious push-pull internal conflict that we experience when we're trying to decide if we want to act on a tempting opportunity. Bat Sheva Marcus, the clinical director of Maze Women's Health in New York City, describes it as:

> It's the "should I or shouldn't I" tantalizing, incredibly sexy part of our psyche. On the one hand, he/she is just not a suitable partner. On the other hand? WOW. We've all been there. People might also experience it with specific sex acts rather than specific partners. "I don't know . . . that (fill in the blank) feels too kinky/scary/edgy to me . . . and yet, it also seems so DAMN HOT" . . . precisely because those things can't necessarily be separated! We each face different ambivalences. It can be as simple as LEAVING THE LIGHTS ON!! It can be as simple as MASTURBATING if you feel guilty about it. It can be as simple as fantasizing about something/someone else.[7]

Think back to when you were in high school: sitting on your bed on a Saturday night, knowing that you were not supposed to be out after 10 pm but also mindful of the fact that your parents are already asleep and it would be just so easy to slip out the back door and meet up with your friends. The tension between the thrill of getting away with something and the fear of getting caught is the essence of violating prohibitions. The way that you feel all tingly and anxious and more than a little bit excited, in that space between recognizing the possibility and making your choice, is where overcoming ambivalence lives. Whatever choice you make—choosing to stay home rather than sneak out, leaving the lights on in the bedroom, or something even more daring—represents a step taken to claim your sexual and relational power. Some ways that you can overcome ambivalence without feeling pressured or coerced include:

- Give yourself time to make up your mind. Often when our partner is asking for something, it can feel like we need to make a quick decision or risk letting them down. Don't forget that patience, denial, and edging are common forms of play within BDSM. Allow yourself the space to think through your options without assuming that a delay means letting your partner down. Ask your partner to think creatively about how to reframe this time for processing into something that feels comfortable and maybe even playful for them.

- Spend time fantasizing about the request. It may seem strange at first to play around with someone else's fantasy, but doing so (especially during solo self-pleasure times) can allow you to imagine a scenario in which their request fits within your comfort zone. As a bonus, the act of letting your brain connect physical pleasure with the idea that you're considering can move the needle from ambivalence toward action.

- Break down the notion into its respective sensory pieces. We often use pro and con lists when trying to decide, but these often prove too "rational" and pragmatic to be useful when working to overcome sexual ambivalence. Plus, "It would make them happy" often outweighs the multiple equally important drawbacks that someone might identify for themselves! Instead, try to make a list of the feelings a particular scenario might evoke for you, both physical and emotional, and consider whether some combination of these might be positive experiences for you. A suggested tickling scene, for example, might make you feel playful, silly, tingly, youthful, overwhelmed, short of breath, aching, or out of control. Do the potential good feelings outweigh the possible bad feelings? How does that inform your decision-making process?

- Consider who it is you're trying to please. Would saying yes make your partner happy? Would saying yes make *you* happy? Does the idea of saying yes make you feel guilty, as if your parents would be ashamed? Are you making choices that are aligned with your spiritual values? You are always allowed to make whatever decision is best for you. Overcoming ambivalence doesn't automatically translate into "Do the thing!" It means making the decision that is best for *you*. Give yourself permission to center your wants, needs, and desires in your decision-making process.

Shared Experimentation

Fox: We are both professional and educated go-getters that tend to spread ourselves thin burning the candle on both ends at times. We both love hard but differ in our love languages. Stephanie prefers words of affirmation and physical touch, where I prefer a show-me-don't-tell-me approach and physical touch. I'm more experienced in nonmonogamy, and with that comes self-confidence, self-awareness, and a steadfast approach to it all. Stephanie is still learning herself in all this and it's both beautiful and scary at times to watch her growth.

Stephanie: I have always been sexually inquisitive but didn't know much about this lifestyle until I met Fox. The way he described his lifestyle captivated me from the start and opened my mind to things I never thought were possible. You can't stop feelings or control them, and that is scary for many. Many in the beginning try to ignore their feelings. We say don't! Listen to your feelings, process them, and then process them with your partner. Feelings are okay, and they can become quite sexy at times. Learn to understand your feelings and teach your partner about them and vice versa. The more we know, the easier and more inviting it becomes.

Fox: There are so many variables that there truly is something for everyone in any way they see fit that is consensual, ethical, and lawful. You don't know what you don't know, and there's no way you fully know yourself when you begin this journey—and that's beautiful. Don't be afraid of the unknown. Allow it to excite you and drive you.

Stephanie: Raw and open communication! Kink is successful because you choose to be open about everything, no matter the topic, even lust for another person(s). It encourages you to advocate for yourself: your needs, wants, desires, and more. It also encourages you to listen to your partner's as well and share them with each other without fear of reaction or judgment. Knowing what your partner is thinking or feeling really builds a certain trust not found in monogamy alone, even when it hurts your feelings. It encourages absolute honesty between each other if you want to continue this style of relationships and not hurt each other.

Fox: Through your love, trust, and communication you tend to adapt a deeper connection, love, and understanding for your partner. You encourage their freedom and that builds compersion (the vicarious joy we feel in knowing that our partner is happy). I tend to find myself loving Stephanie's growth and connection with others. It helps me find the love to encourage her more and more in her pursuits.

Stephanie: If you and your partner are not having hard conversations that make your stomach turn, then you're not really talking. It gets better and easier, we promise you, but you gotta go where society tells you not to. Only there will you find your true self to share with your partner. And hell yes, that is scary. We all fear that our loved one(s) would cringe, run, vomit at the inner dirty thoughts we have. What if instead of that reaction, you got a high five, a smile, a kiss, or a slap on the butt with a kinky wink from your partner?! Let your dirty freak flag fly and the right partner will hoist it up higher for you while you are busy getting your freak on. Be 100 percent—yes, 100 percent—open about your lust, kinks, fetishes, thoughts, needs, wants, and hard no's. It is oh-so worth it, though, to know you can be yourself without fear of judgment. Wow is it empowering!

Fox: Remember that it's not a race! Only move as physically or emotionally fast as the slowest person in the relationship. Encouragement is good, but make sure it's not selfish in nature or you endanger your relationship. Never allow others to push you faster than comfortable. Always be safe emotionally, physically, and sexually in everything you do.

—Stephanie, 40, and Fox, 44

Building Trust Through Play

One of our primary ways of connecting to others and building relationships is with playfulness. From the game of peekaboo we almost instinctively strike up with the baby ahead of us in the grocery checkout line, to the structured team-building activities of the business world, we are wired to bond through play. Play is physical. It is sensory. It is imaginative. Play allows us to bring our full selves into a specific place and moment, and to share that experience with those who are with us. It's no wonder, then, why most kinky people describe their scenes and sexual encounters as "play." Consciously or not, we bring many elements of those past playground games with us into our intimate lives, using the social and emotional tools of play to heighten our sexual and relational connections.

BLIND MAN'S BLUFF: Sensory deprivation is one of the most common forms of BDSM play. From vanilla couples looking to spice up their sex lives to lifestyle BDSM players, the use of blindfolds, gags, and other devices that limit one or more of the senses are very popular. We fail to realize just how reliant we are on our sight, speech and hearing until we experience the absence of them. Experimenting with limiting our senses can turn an otherwise ordinary sexual encounter into something surprisingly novel.

COPS AND ROBBERS: Children are infinitely creative in finding ways to weave restraints, struggle, and captivity into their play. Whether it takes the form of cops and robbers, pirates and captives, playing army, or imagining themselves as princess-prisoners being rescued by valiant knights, much early imagination play includes elements of "bondage" that kinky adults might recognize and connect to later in life. Whether locked in a closet, tied up with jump ropes, or guarded by others, they love to act out these themes through play. In adulthood, bringing restraints into the bedroom is another incredibly common way to enhance intimacy. The stereotypical fuzzy handcuffs are just one of a vast spectrum of restraint devices that allow partners to play with different positions, explore sex within creative constraints, and experience the fun and frustration that comes from restricting their various movements.

MOTHER MAY I/SIMON SAYS: Giving and receiving direction is a key element in many power-exchange relationships. Whether the leading partner is issuing a command to be followed or imposing a prohibition to be avoided, the following partner's role is to obey to the best of their ability. Those who enjoy power exchange find comfort and security in knowing what the expectations are, when to act, and when to refrain. Our interest in playing with authority in this way may show up in the myriad of playground games that focus on giving and following orders. One of my favorite homework activities to give to my sex therapy clients is to play Simon Says in the bedroom. Reframing direction-giving as a game can be incredibly helpful in helping partners find their voices in the bedroom. For others, carrying this over into their daily lives outside of the bedroom (through some form of power-exchange agreement) can be a powerful way to enhance their relationship communication and their understanding of their partner's needs and desires.

THE FLOOR IS LAVA: When we think of BDSM and kink, we usually think of clearly defined hierarchical roles with specific rules and restrictions. We imagine a structured, orderly lifestyle where there's a place for everyone and everyone knows their place. And this is certainly true for many power-exchange relationships. But within this paradigm there exists a form of power play that delights in ambiguity: predicament play. In the same way that the Floor Is Lava sets a simple goal for the players but then imposes restrictions that increase the difficulty, predicament play asks the submissive partner to do something rather simple and adds in elements that make the process of complying uncomfortable, arousing, or frustrating to achieve:

Predicament play refers to a variety of sadomasochistic/kinky activities in which there is a particular set of physical parameters (e.g. through rope, other restraints, and/or other devices) which simultaneously encourage and/or discourage different and mutually exclusive responses. The person in the predicament is faced with having to choose among, and lean into or away from, various painful or pleasurable or strange stimuli. Predicaments often involve a slow-burn, building up of intensity, from something that is set in motion initially and then becomes more difficult/painful/overwhelming over the ensuing seconds and minutes. Predicament play often appeals to the more creative, quirky, and even ridiculous SM players, bringing out our inner mad-scientist sadists & James Bond escape artist masochists. A predicament could be as complex as a Rube Goldberg machine—or as simple as being forced to stand on one leg until that becomes unbearably painful. Predicaments tend to involve being between a proverbial "rock and a hard place" while trying to figure a way out (even when there's probably no way out—just a choice between one sadistic trap and another).[8]

MONKEY IN THE MIDDLE: I'm going to tell you a secret. I was not a popular kid in grade school. I was one of the nerdy, awkward children that preferred to sit alone and read during recess. As a result, I was bullied mercilessly. This is what comes to mind for me when I think of the game Monkey in the Middle, or as it was often called on the playgrounds of my youth, Keep Away. The goal of this game is quite simple. Two or more people toss an object back and forth over the head of another who stands in between them. The center person simply has to catch it. Easy enough if everyone involved has consented to playing the game. Frustrating and humiliating when the "monkey" did not choose to be placed in the middle. Degradation/humiliation kinks can be hard for folks to wrap their heads around until we reflect on the casual sadism of childhood. For some kinky adults, playing with scenes of degradation/humiliation can be an incredibly intimate, often cathartic, experience. Intimate because we must know our partner incredibly well in order to set a scene that evokes this kind of emotional reaction in them, and cathartic because playing in such a way with someone who cares deeply about our heart and safety can facilitate our ability to reprocess and recontextualize some of our own deepest fears and insecurities. Princess Kali, a dominant and kink educator specializing in erotic humiliation, writes, "Humiliation requires that you tune in to the individual person that you're playing with. There's so much of the mind to explore, and people have such a different approach to their desires that your ability to 'poke at' all of those dark spaces is what makes humiliation play an exciting adventure. . . . What one person finds humiliating, another person might find liberating."[9]

PLAYING HOUSE: Children learn through watching and emulating the world around them. This emulation often occurs during play, which is why play therapy is such an effective intervention for youngsters. Playing house allows children to experiment with taking on different roles and experiencing how each one feels. What does it feel like to be the baby in a family versus the daddy? Is there a difference between being the big sister and being the little brother? Do I have to be a girl to take on the role of Mommy in this imaginary family?

TEA PARTIES: In a similar way, tea parties allow children to explore elements of traditional gender roles, primarily through the clothing and behavior expected of girls and women. Pulling a feather boa and a plastic crown out of the toy box and hosting one's stuffed animals for tea creates another experiential learning opportunity: What does it feel like to be "fancy," to be proper, to be a gracious host, to be a refined lady? Each of these experiences inform the young person's understanding of who they are, how they fit in the world, and the social roles that feel most comfortable for them. It's rather sad that this imagination play is one of the first things we put aside as we move into adolescence and then on to adulthood. Thankfully, for many adults, this continues through their practice of BDSM and kink!

As we've already discussed, gender presentation and role performance can be an enjoyable element of BDSM play for people across the gender spectrum. Having a space as adults to dress up (whether in leather catsuits or pastel onesies) and feel sexy, "fancy," seductive, or simply our most authentic selves for a brief moment in time is a delightful experience that most of us who have aged out of our prom years don't get to have regularly. Likewise, playing with ideas of polite, proper society can bring another layer to our relationships and our socialization both in and out of the bedroom. A sadistic dominant in a business suit may delight in having their submissive partner prepare and serve a formal tea service for them each afternoon. The submissive's attention to detail in preparing an orderly arrangement of sandwiches and a properly prepared pot of tea becomes a tangible show of affection and a desire to please. Likewise, the Leather Daddy (a title claimed by people of all genders) might savor the site of their slave boi carefully trimming and lighting their cigars before kneeling beside their chair and silently holding their ashtray aloft. Their boi's willingness to remain silent and available signals their willingness to place the Leather Daddy's comfort ahead of their own, even if they do not interact with them beyond the taps of their cigar against their dish. The kinky ability to step in and out of wardrobes and roles, to assume an identity for an evening or create a dynamic that lasts a lifetime, is one of the most powerful ways kinky people use play to build trust.

PLAYING PRETEND: In the same way that children play-act adulthood and experiment with taking on different cultural and gendered roles, so too do many youngsters enjoy pretending that they are something else altogether! In second grade, my small friend group spent every recess deeply absorbed in the faerie community that existed only in our minds. We would run and laugh, pretending to fly and cast spells, calling one another by the flower-themed faerie names that could only be acknowledged within the sacred world of the playground. In another corner of the same schoolyard were the children who took on the personas of animals. We faeries flew past a variety of tigers, elephants, monkeys, and more. Beyond this invisible zoo were the children who spent their recesses exploring the world of machines: pretend tractors and dump trucks, anthropomorphic airplanes. The playground contained a universe of imaginary identities. This was not play that let us preview our future adult roles. It was an opportunity to ignore these prescribed roles altogether and pretend that we could (as parents and teachers promised) really, truly grow up to be anything we wanted to be—even a faerie, a puppy, or a train.

As we discussed briefly in chapter 3, BDSM play opens up the doors to a wide variety of role-play both realistic and fantastical. The ability to embody a persona that isn't our everyday reality can feel freeing and relaxing, playful and connective. There is a vast body of research on the benefits of play therapy for children and adults, and the ability to set aside the performance pressure that so many of us experience in everyday life to simply *play* with one another can feel as restorative as it is silly. Some kinky people use their power-exchange relationships for this purpose. They don't necessarily live a 24/7 lifestyle, but they enjoy assuming the roles of leader and follower for a brief period of "real make-believe." Sometimes there are layers of playing pretend woven into the kinky scene. They might take on the role of a beloved pet (often a kitten, puppy, or pony) and its handler. They might return to some of the activities they enjoyed in childhood and play-act a younger person who indulges in coloring books and cartoons, stickers and storybooks, with a partner who takes on the role of caregiver.

RED ROVER/LONDON BRIDGE: Do you remember springtime in elementary school, when the weather was clear and warm enough for your gym teacher to move the class outdoors? One popular game for days like these was Red Rover, wherein the class was divided into two teams that stood holding hands in lines facing one another. Each team would take turns calling out "Red rover, red rover, send *Jackie* right over!" When their name was called, it was Jackie's turn to run pell-mell across the span toward the wall of other children as fast as they could in order to break through their clasped hands. If they managed to break the line, they "stole" one of the other team members back to their own team's line. If not? They joined the end of the chain of children. It was a physical game, predicated on power and brute force, that often left the players laughing with their butts in the dirt. Red Rover stands out as one of the few "violent" playground games that many children were allowed to play. And for the most part, we loved it.

For younger children, this joyful physicality was often experienced during toddler games of London Bridge. In this game, two children face each other and clasp hands, raising them both above their heads to form an arch. The other children line up and take turns passing beneath their raised hands until the song comes to an end, at which point the last child through is "captured" when the bridged arms fall to surround them. From there, the bridge children swing their arms, rocking the captured child back and forth, buffeting them against the locked arms before laughingly releasing them to rejoin the line and start again. The common theme in both London Bridge and Red Rover is the idea of controlled roughhousing, joyful aggression, and a consensual approach to behaviors that might, in another context, be experienced as bullying.

For many kinky people, this notion of consensual, playful, exuberant aggression is present in how they engage with BDSM play. Some might indulge in what is known as "rough body play," such as punching large-muscle areas of the thighs, buttocks, and back. Others might love watching wrestling scenes, where attractive men or women roll and tussle for dominance on the gym mat before the pinned party submits to the winner's desires. Still others might identify as "primal" players and get off on the thrill of chasing their partner around, wrestling them to the ground, and "forcing" sexual surrender, much like wolves might take down a deer in the forest. To the outside observer, rough body play can look scary, even criminal. The idea of overpowering someone and dominating them physically before sex might feel similar to assault if one doesn't know what they're seeing. However, just like in our childhood games of Red Rover, the brute force used in these scenes is a toy, not a weapon. The goal is not to injure each other or to coerce an unwilling person into sexual activity they genuinely oppose. The goal is a London Bridge–style tumble—a playful roughing-up that allows everyone involved to test their mettle, prove their strength, and make the other person really *earn* their erotic reward.

As mentioned earlier, one of my favorite childhood games was Mad Libs. My friends and I spent hours creating silly stories (and learning the parts of speech!) by filling in the blanks with ridiculous nouns, adverbs, and adjectives. My Fantasy Fill-In is a more serious version of that slumber-party staple. You don't have to fill it out all at once. You may even fill it out differently at different times or on different days. That's wonderful! There is no right or wrong here—it's simply a framework for you to think about what you want most from an intimate experience. Do one alone as a tool of self-reflection. Do it together with your partner and then compare notes. Use it to help find the words to think about—and ask for—what you want in a way that feels natural and safe. You can download and print this worksheet at stefanigoerlich.com/with-sprinkles-on-top-worksheets.html#/.

My Fantasy Fill-In

When we have sex, I need _____.
My focus tonight is (is/is not) on having an orgasm. I want to feel
_____, and one of the best ways to get me there is to
_____ my _____, to say
_____ to me while _____. I
love the feel of _____ and would love to include
that in our play together. When you _____, it
makes me feel _____, and I really want that to be a
part of our time together. On the other hand, I don't want to ____
_____ because it makes me feel
_____ and that's not what I want this time. I want
you to know that when I watch you _____,
I get really _____, and that is one of my favorite
parts of being with you. I love seeing your _____ when
we touch each other, and I really love your _____ in
my _____. Sometimes I like to imagine _____
_____, and I think it would be
really hot if we could play around more with that idea together. When
you call me _____, it feeds that fantasy for me and
my body _____. I think it would be fun if you
_____ me on the _____. I really
want you to be _____ with me. And afterward,
I want to _____ while you _____.
What do you think? Can I tempt you tonight?

MORE TO READ ON THIS TOPIC

A Billion Wicked Thoughts: What the Internet Tells Us about Sexual Relationships

Ogi Ogas and Sai Gaddam

Different Loving: The World of Sexual Dominance and Submission

Gloria G. Brame, William D. Brame, and Jon Jacobs

Tell Me What You Want: The Science of Sexual Desire and How It Can Help You Improve Your Sex Life

Justin Lehmiller

6

What's Normal, Anyway?

In my work with clients, I often ask them to tell me what they want for themselves and their partners, what their ideal resolution to whatever challenge has brought them to therapy might be. The answer, regardless of the issue, is nearly universal: "I just want to be normal."

"I want to desire sex as much as normal people do."

"I want to have a normal amount of sex."

"I just want a plain, old, normal kinky lifestyle."

"I just want a normal relationship with a normal person."

The problem is that we use *normal* as if it were a unit of measurement or an objective term. In reality (as we've already discussed), what is normal depends entirely on the time, place, and culture that we live in. By way of an example, let's look at that *other* subject that, along with sex, we're taught not to discuss in polite company: religion. What kind of answers would I get if I asked my clients how they "normally" celebrated the spring holiday with their families?

My clients from Eastern Europe might tell me they're spending time using beeswax and red and black dyes to carefully make elaborate pysanky designs on hollowed-out eggshells. My clients from Western Europe might share that they're planning on walking the stations of the cross before taking home palm fronds to weave into Brigid's crosses to hang in the home. Latin American clients might recall the last time they visited their home village to watch devoted members of their community be literally nailed to a cross in order to align themselves with Christ's suffering. Clients from the southern

147

United States may share that they've set their alarms for 3 am so that they can get to sunrise service, where they will raise their hands and shout "Hallelujah" as the choir sings. Some of my clients might say that they don't buy into the whole "religion thing" but that they still take their kids to sit on the lap of a mall employee wearing a bunny costume. And still others will look at me, smile, and say that they'll be purging their house of all leavened products so they can host the second-night seder for their friends.

You might see your own spiritual observance reflected here or you might celebrate the springtime in a completely different way. So, tell me, which of these answers tells us what is normal?

The same is true when we talk about sexuality and relationships. "Normal" isn't a destination; it's a spectrum. What is normal for you—from libido levels to sexual frequency, from kinky play to how we define monogamy—can and will vary from person to person. Each answer will fall somewhere on the spectrum, of course, but there's very rarely a cause for us to call something abnormal or incorrect. There's only what feels right for your body and what works best for your relationship . . . and just like celebrating the holidays, there may be some common answers, but there's no such thing as normal.

HOW MUCH SEX IS NORMAL?

This is perhaps the most common question I am asked when my clients first begin sex therapy. Most people, after all, want to feel as if their bodies are working "right," that their needs are "reasonable," and that they are demanding neither too much nor too little from their partner. One of the first conversations that we have together is around the notion that normal is itself a subjective thing based on several variables that combine into unique combinations for each partnership I work with. Even if I were working with identical twins who were the exact same gender, age, and sexual orientation and from the same family, culture, and location? Their respective partners would *not* share these common traits, which would result in two very different, highly personalized relationship experiences for each sibling. In other words, the cliché is true: normal really is just a setting on the dryer! We can take a quick look at what the averages look like across the various experiences we bring with us into our intimate relationships—not because they are a standard we need to meet but so we can see where, quite often, we fall well within the "range of normal" and where we don't. We don't often deviate quite so much. Having a basis of comparison (not a benchmark to achieve) can be reassuring in that respect.

By Age

The idea that younger people report having more sex than those who are older probably isn't a shocking piece of news to you. After all, the average age of first intercourse is 16.8 years for men and 17.2 for women.[1] Most of us carry cultural messages that tell us that sexuality is for the young and nubile and that once the blush of youth fades, we put the erotic on the shelf, alongside our high school letterman's jacket and our childhood baby shoes. It can be a pleasant surprise, then, to learn just how active our intimate lives tend to be even as we age! According to the Kinsey Institute, 28 percent of Americans age forty-five and older report that they had sexual intercourse at least once per week in the last six months, while 22 percent reported that they had masturbated at least once per week. Another 40 percent of folks age forty-five and older have sex at least once per month.[2] This number stays fairly consistent even as we enter our retirement years, where 40 percent of folks between the ages of sixty-five and eighty report maintaining physical intimacy with their partners.[3] While those numbers decline as we move into old age, one in four people between the ages of seventy-six and eighty state that they are still sexually active![4] What do these statistics mean in terms of actual numbers of sexual encounters? The Kinsey Institute has an answer for us there too:

> Specifically, the team behind the research found that people between the ages of 18 and 29 are having the most sex, with an average of 112 sex sessions per year (which translates, roughly, to twice a week). Folks between the ages of 30 and 39 have sex 1.6 times per week (or 86 times per year). Those between the ages of 40 and 49 engage in sexual acts about 69 times per year.[5]

By Gender

Most men report having partnered sex two to four times per month, although as we've already discussed, these numbers vary a bit based on age. Only 6.1 percent of men report having sex more than four times per week.[6] When it comes to solo sex, approximately one in four men report masturbating "a few times per week to monthly,"[7] and the majority told researchers they had masturbated at least once in the last year.[8] On the other hand, one in five women in that same study told researchers they'd masturbated in the past month, and 40 percent said they'd engaged in solo sex at least once in the last year.[9] This is in addition to the "weekly or more" sexual activity that the majority of women reported having with their partners.[10] You might be reading this section wondering what "normal" looks like for folks who fall outside of the cis male-female binary. Unfortunately there has not been much research done yet on the intimate lives of gender-fluid or nonbinary individuals. This is an important area for social and medical researchers to be aware of so that we can start to fill in the gaps in our knowledge of human sexuality and relationships.

By Relationship Status

Another relationship myth that many of us hear is the idea of "marital bed death"—the belief that getting married signals the death knell of our sex lives. The old ball and chain, who keeps her husband from sowing his wild oats, is a common joke at bachelor parties and wedding receptions. But is this trope supported by the data? Survey says . . . *no*! Married couples and dating couples have roughly the same amount of sex: 1.2 times per week versus 1.1 times per week, respectively. Single folks report having sex .3 times per week (or roughly once per month). Interestingly, couples who are not married but are living together have sex approximately 1.6 times per week.[11]

Approximately 20 percent of married couples and 70 percent of couples in committed dating relationships will encounter infidelity at some point during the life of their relationship; the percentage, by age, of folks who admitted to cheating on their partner was relatively consistent (ranging from 17–21 percent) across age groups,[12] although men are more likely to cheat than women.[13] Oddly enough, people who engage in affairs do not necessarily have more sex than their faithful peers: 91 percent of all women and 77 percent of all men admit to having an emotional (but not necessarily physical) affair; while 53 percent of women and 72 percent of men reported engaging in a one-night stand.[14] These encounters, combined with cybersex/online affairs (40 percent of women and 30.6 percent of men[15]) tell us that infidelity, when it occurs, does not necessarily result in more physical intimacy for those involved. And infidelity does not necessarily mean the relationship itself is failing! One private detective agency released a report detailing their findings after years of being hired to catch cheating partners. They found "56% of men and 34% of women who commit infidelity rate their marriages as happy or very happy. This makes the reason people cheat a little harder to dissect and comprehend."[16]

By Orientation

According to Justin Lehmiller, men in committed relationships report having sex about seven times per month with their primary partner, regardless of their sexual orientation. More than half of both gay and straight men reported being sexually satisfied.[17] Conversely, women in lesbian relationships report having sex less often than their peers in heterosexual relationships, with 42 percent of gay women reporting they have sex zero to one time per month compared to just 15 percent of straight women.[18] Megan Martin theorizes women in same-sex relationships may have less sex because the intimate moments they do share are longer in duration and more sexually satisfying.[19] In fact, research shows that lesbian women are more likely to report behaviors associated with romantic intimacy such as gentle kissing, oral sex, sex lasting longer than thirty minutes, and hearing "I love you" from their partner during sex.[20]

"Both gay and straight couples tend to have sex less frequently in long-term relationships. A 'sex rate' of three times per week for gay male couples in the first two years of a relationship is almost 70 percent. It drops to less than 50 percent for straight couples and to about 33 percent for lesbian couples."[21] These numbers don't include folks in open or ethically nonmonogamous relationships. "Approximately 89% reported being in monogamous partnerships, 4% reported open relationships (what some call consensual nonmonogamy), and 8% reported being supposedly monogamous (what some call nonconsensual non-monogamy)," so there may be some increase in sexual frequency where there is also an increase in the number of sexual partners.[22]

By Race

Some of the most pernicious and harmful stereotypes are those that try to connect a person's race to their sexual behaviors. These mistaken beliefs have resulted in racial animosity directed toward Black men perceived as sexually aggressive and dangerous, the hypersexualization of women from many racial and ethnic groups that results in girls being perceived as more sexually mature and developmentally advanced than they are, and myths about the bodies of Asian men and their desirability as partners. The data does not support these biases. Researchers "failed to detect any significant differences across racial groups" when it came to sexual frequency.[23]

Asexuality/Demisexuality

We can't talk about sexual orientation without touching on the concept of asexuality, which can itself be a spectrum ranging from *entirely sex revulsed* to *experiencing sexual attraction to others only when an emotional bond occurs (often called demisexuality)* with many points in between. The Asexual Visibility and Education Network (AVEN) defines asexuality as "someone who does not experience sexual attraction or an intrinsic desire to have sexual relationships."[24] According to the Kinsey Institute, roughly .5–1 percent of Americans are estimated to be asexual.[25] The term used for folks who experience sexual attraction or who desire sexual relationships is *allosexual*. These two terms are often abbreviated to "ace" and "allo," respectively.

Often clients will ask me how they can tell the difference between being somewhere on the ace spectrum versus just having low libido/low desire. There is no empirical measurement for sexuality, of course. We can't analyze a blood sample and declare someone asexual any more than we can separate heterosexual blood from bisexual blood. I typically tell my clients that low libido only becomes a clinical problem *if and when* it becomes a problem for them. If someone is happy and content without experiencing sexual attraction and desire? They may choose to self-identify as being somewhere on the spectrum of asexuality and build happy and fulfilling relationships that don't include sexual activities. If, on the other hand, this absence of desire represents a change in their usual physiological and emotional responses, or if it causes them distress to not desire sexual contact? There are some common medical and physiological reasons why someone might experience diminished or absent desire, and we would explore these possibilities together.

That is not to say that asexual people *never* engage in sexual activities either alone or with a partner. Angela Chen, the author of *ACE: What Asexuality Reveals about Desire, Society, and the Meaning of Sex*, writes,

To the best I can tell, sexual attraction is the desire to have sex with a specific person, for physical reasons. Sexual attraction can be instantaneous and involuntary: a heightened awareness, a physical alertness, combined with mental wanting . . . Fair enough. Aces don't experience this. Aces can still find people beautiful, have a libido, masturbate, and seek out porn. Aces can enjoy sex and like kink and be in relationships of all kinds . . . Sexual attraction, then, is horniness towards or caused by a specific person. It is the desire to be sexual with that partner—libido with a target. . . . And just as people have different sex drives, they also experience different levels of sexual attraction. Some aces have a libido and some don't, but we all share the lack of sexual attraction, and most of us have a low desire for partnered sex.[26]

Demisexual Desire

I was raised in a very repressive religious environment: Anything beyond kissing before marriage was wrong. I wasn't allowed to dress like other teens because it was seen as provocative. In fact, I attributed my lack of attraction to that for ages.

When my spouse and I *did* have sex before marriage, I was so disappointed and heartbroken in fact to discover that that wasn't the case. They're an attentive, loving partner and I felt betrayed . . . not by them but by all of my upbringing that implied that once you "do it," you'll unlock like some sort of sexual being.

I love the concept of sex, and romance especially, but in reality it's a bit like those folks who want to homestead and then buy a farm and really quickly realize that the reality of it is pretty intense.

My partner is bi. They were up front about this from day one. When I told them I was asexual, they responded, "Yeah. No kidding. Kinda figured," and they laughed.

On the other hand, it honestly didn't click until recently that my partner is *very* submissive. A friend of ours pointed it out to me after spending some time with us. After that conversation, I essentially tried a few mild Dom power moves and they were putty in my hands. It was sweet to see. Because they enjoyed it. And while I am not a huge fan of the actual act of sex, seeing my partner enjoy themselves makes it worth it. Now that I know this, and when I'm in the mood, I can much more easily make them happier. It's like we've discovered some new sort of recipe. It's kinda fun actually! I'm a very dominant, bossy person. So, I basically keep doing what I've been doing but with more intentionality. I make sure to use aftercare as well as continual check-ins to make sure they're still cool with what we're doing.

You've got to have an open mind and a few ideas and curiosities themselves, beyond the limits of just P-in-V sex; if you're patient, you may get to discover them together. But going at their pace is key. Sexual contact is already not something I necessarily *love* to experience, but if you find the common ground, you may still have struggles but they won't seem as impossible to overcome. For example, I'm more than willing to edge my partner, bringing them close to orgasm over and over again, letting them feel completely within my control, before finishing them off with a hand job. That's something I'm totally comfortable doing as a demisexual because it requires very little of me—I don't even need to take off my clothes! But it gives them the feeling of surrender and domination, as well as the sexual release, that I know they want.

I wish I'd known about my sexuality and how they're submissive sooner. I think a lot of fights in the beginning of our relationship wouldn't have happened, because they have a hell of a time saying no to anything. I've only *once* seen them have a hard no. So knowing this would have enabled me to ask in a different way that wouldn't entail them saying no directly, because that led to a lot of resentment when we were first married. Now I approach our conflicts in a way that lets them have a "submissive" response to me: either "If it would make you happy" for yes or "Not unless you want to" for no.

—Hazel, 36

WHAT'S NORMAL TO FEEL DURING SEX?

Remember those romance novels that we discussed a few chapters back? Those books, along with other erotic material such as movies and porn, are the first (and often only) education many folks get about sexual pleasure. The linear, procreation-focused sex-ed classes certainly never stop to answer the question "But what does sex *feel* like?" Even within those bodice-ripping pages, the descriptions are often so hyperbolic and symbolic (fireworks! dancing goddesses! crashing oceans!) that many of my clients come to therapy not quite sure of what "successful" sex should feel like . . . or whether they've ever had that experience for themselves. They want to know what is normal to feel during sex. And, as with most things, the answer is "It depends."

Pleasure

Laurie Mintz, educator, pleasure activist, and author of *Becoming Cliterate*, describes a phenomenon she calls the pleasure gap: the differences between how often men and women experience orgasm during partnered sex. In her work, she noted some fascinating facts about who experiences pleasure during sex, and how often:

- Only 57 percent of women say they reach orgasm "most or every time" during sex . . . compared to 95 percent of men![27]

- Gay women have significantly more orgasms than straight women.[28]

- Women have more orgasms through masturbation than via partner sex.[29]

It's not that women are less capable of achieving orgasm; skin (for all genders) contains over one hundred nerve endings per square inch, and the clitoris specifically has even more! The clitoris contains twice the number of nerve endings as the penis, in a space roughly twenty times smaller, which creates an opportunity for intense sensation for those who seek it out. Most people of all genders are capable of pleasure during sex.[30] For many, barring injury or disability, that pleasure takes the form of physical sensations. For most, there is also emotional pleasure as well. The body responds to these sensations through increased heart rate and blood flow, which causes the skin to flush, the muscles to tingle, and the genitals (in all genders) to swell and become more sensitive.

PHYSICAL

Sex researchers William Masters and Virginia Johnson were among the first to observe the biology of sex as it happened. Through their work, they described a four-stage cycle of sexual arousal: excitement, plateau, orgasm, and resolution. Excitement often occurs during what's commonly called foreplay—the touching, kissing, teasing, and caressing that offers moments of varied physical sensations and emotional connection to your partner. During the plateau phase (which often, but not always, corresponds with penetration either by a penis, a toy, or fingers), the genitals become hyper-sensitive and actually retract a bit from contact—the testicles draw up into the scrotum or the clitoris retracts under the clitoral hood. These intense sensations can cause muscle contraction; spasms in the feet, hands, and face; and a feeling of full-body pressure or tension as blood pressures rise. For many people, the plateau phase reaches its peak with orgasm, when the genital-pelvic muscles (in all genders) begin to repeatedly contract and release. This spurs ejaculation from the penis and a sensation of tightness and relaxation in the uterus.[31] What Masters and Johnson called the resolution period, most of us just call the "afterglow," a time where partners rest and recover, enjoying the sense of closeness their proximity affords, as their skin cools and their heart rate and blood pressure come down. For some bodies, the intensity of the sensation they experience at the edge of the plateau heading toward an orgasm is so intense that they pull back, choosing instead to prolong the milder but still deeply satisfying sensations of extended plateau rather than focusing on the short intensity of an orgasm, and that's a valid choice! Others love that intensity and will cultivate as many orgasms as their bodies can afford—an equally valid choice!

EMOTIONAL

Believe it or not, the emotional connection that we experience (whether we call it love, mutual attraction, or something in between) is also rooted in our biology. When we spend time engaging in intimate physical contact with another person (with or without penetrative intercourse), our brain responds to these physical sensations in a way that directly influences our moods and emotions. In other words, our hormones are impacting not just *what* we feel but *how* we feel as well:

- Oxytocin is released throughout the sexual encounter, while our bodies are most actively engaged with our partners. Often called the "cuddle hormone," oxytocin is associated with forming feelings of trust, affection, intimacy, and bonding. Oxytocin is also released during nonsexual intimate moments as well, such as when a mother nurses her newborn or when you spend time gazing into your beloved's eyes.

- Vasopressin, another hormone associated with intimacy and bonding, is also released during sex. Interestingly, vasopressin also reduces pain sensations in the body, which may explain why some BDSM activities that look incredibly painful to the outside observer are not only tolerated but enjoyed by those involved in a sensory play scene.[32]

- Dopamine, which is responsible for our feelings of pleasure, desire, and motivation, is released during orgasm. "Some refer to dopamine as a 'pleasure' chemical—though research has shown it offers us much more than just a good time. It's really more of a learning chemical, helping to take notice of rewards like food and sex, and figure out how to get more of them."[33] This physiological learning response may be why some folks approach sex as a reward for "good behavior" in their relationships—a mindset that can be incredibly frustrating or incredibly useful, depending upon the partners!

- After orgasm, the brain releases serotonin, which is related to relaxation and positive moods. Serotonin can also make us sleepy, which may explain (along with the physical exertion of higher pulses and contracting muscles) why so many of us want a good nap after sex!

This is not to say that sex, or sexual play, must be an emotional experience for you. After all, our hormones may provoke certain physiological responses in the body, but it remains up to the mind to interpret and give meaning to those reactions. Sex educator Lauren Brim reminds us that "as social creatures, we are designed to bond through a variety of activities, but the sex often creates a sense that we *should* form a relationship with the person because society has designated that as part of our social sexual script."[34] For many people, sexual intimacy is a key building block in how they form and maintain deep relationships. For others, it's a sensory activity that feels good in the moment, much like a gourmet meal or a great foot massage, but doesn't carry the emotional weight that it might for others. Whether you prefer to focus on creating opportunities for sensory enjoyment (with or without orgasm) during sex, whether you prioritize the way intimacy makes you feel emotionally, or whether you want a mix of both somatic and romantic connection, you are in charge of deciding what you want sex to feel like for you.

Pain

For some folks, the answer to "What do you want sex to feel like?" is a complicated one. There are many reasons why sexual intimacy is not enjoyable for them, ranging from chronic health conditions, to negative messages about sex that they internalized growing up, to traumatic experiences that have caused sex to be something fearful rather than pleasurable. And then there are others for whom discomfort, and even pain, is a part of how they experience pleasure, which can feel complicated to explain to someone who isn't wired in that same way. For many of my clients and readers, for better or worse, pain is a normal part of their experiences of intimacy.

PHYSICAL

Sex and intimacy are rooted in our experiences of the body. Beginning with our earlier conversation about the ways in which our physical selves influence our emotional selves via hormones, we can't have a conversation about what sex feels like without acknowledging the ways in which variations in our body can influence those feelings. There are a myriad of injuries, chronic conditions, and bodily states that impact if and how our bodies receive sensation, including:

- Vaginismus is an involuntary condition wherein the vaginal muscles constrict, making penetration very painful, if possible at all.

- Peyronie's disease causes scar tissue to develop on the penis, causing a bend in the shaft of the penis, and results in pain during erections as well as limits sexual functioning.

- Endometriosis is when uterine tissue grows outside of the uterus, often in the ovaries or fallopian tubes.

- Infections (such as bacterial vaginosis or yeast), pelvic inflammatory disease, as well as sexually transmitted infections such as gonorrhea and chlamydia can cause tissue irritation or blisters (in the case of herpes). While many men with these conditions are asymptomatic, they can transmit infections to their partners who might experience symptoms that make intercourse (or even genital touching) uncomfortable.

- Eczema, lichen sclerosus, and other skin conditions cause irritation, rashes, and blistered or broken skin that is painful to the touch.

- Hemorrhoids are swollen blood vessels, which are sometimes externally visible, that can occur in the anal area due to childbirth, pressure from chronic constipation, or even sex. Hemorrhoid pain can be exacerbated by sexual contact, which naturally makes intimacy uncomfortable as well.

- Cancer can have significant impact on the sexual functioning of all genders. Necessary treatments may result in difficult erections, vaginal dryness, nausea, or pain—all of which can feel like barriers to intimacy.

- Scar tissue from routine surgeries or other injuries often is more fibrous and not as flexible as unbroken skin. This can result in discomfort and pain during certain positions or activities.

- Nerve or spinal injuries can result in conflicting symptoms, depending upon the cause or condition. Some injuries may reduce or eliminate sensation entirely, leaving a person unable to feel sensations at all. On the other hand, degenerative nerve conditions might have the opposite effect, rendering them so incredibly sensitive to touch that any sensation at all feels painful.

- Irritable bowel syndrome (IBS) symptoms can make sex both physically and psychologically uncomfortable. It can also impact sexual performance, with one study finding that men with IBS were more likely to develop erectile dysfunction compared to their peers without the disorder.[35]

This is far from a comprehensive list, of course. The important thing to understand is that our understanding of "normal" sex usually assumes that normal equals pain-free. And yet there are dozens of factors that can result in a person's normal day-to-day experience of sexual intimacy being one that includes painful sensations as well as pleasure. For some people with chronic health conditions, embracing painful sensations and choosing to include pain in their sexual play is a way to claim mastery over their chronic health concerns and to reframe something that might feel tragic or hopeless into a tool they have agency over and find benefit from.[36] That's one example of how our psychological mindset can impact our physical experience of pain. Let's look at a few other examples of this mind-body connection.

PSYCHOLOGICAL

Beginning as early as the days we watched Saturday morning cartoons, we are taught that love, sex, romance, and intimacy should be accompanied by the warm-fuzzy feelings of butterflies in the stomach and hearts in our eyes. So many of us are raised with negative messages around our bodies and sexuality—ideas of purity, rules about wardrobe and makeup and what they supposedly say about us, expectations about "appropriate" behavior for girls versus boys . . . all of the ways in which we are socialized to define ourselves and our sexuality according to the understanding of outsiders! And then . . . a switch is flipped and all of a sudden we are supposed to feel those butterflies and leap joyfully into a healthy adult sexual relationship. If only it were so easy.

Unfortunately, guilt and shame are a part of the "normal" sexual experience for many, often due to trauma they've experienced related to their bodies and sexual selves. As the psychotherapist Ruth Cohn writes,

> At the core of trauma is a profound experience of helplessness and of being worthless or insignificant. This is true whether the trauma is a rape or an earthquake. There's no stopping the powerful approaching, overwhelming force. And that force, whatever it is, does not care how the victim feels. Because helplessness is an utterly unbearable human emotion, we will do anything in our power to avoid feeling it. One defense against helplessness is guilt: the irrational belief that "there is something I could have done, I just didn't do it." . . . Guilt is a ready default and is often reinforced by a blaming world. . . .

Shame and guilt are some of the most persistent emotional by-products
of trauma and abuse and can readily evolve into self-hatred and a sense of
integral "badness."[37]

Whether our trauma takes the form of unattainable social expectations, unstable relationships, or sexual abuse, we often internalize these feelings and process them through our sexual selves. This can take the form of what used to be called "frigidity"—shutting down our capacity to give and receive pleasure and maintaining distance both emotionally and physically from our partners. For others, sexuality becomes a cathartic outlet, a way to process their traumatic experiences and emotional pain and to confront them. Proximity, emotionally and physically, to a trusted (or even loved) other who is willing to hold space for us as we challenge these negative emotions, as well as the physical reactions they evoke in our body, can be a deep form of healing. Some BDSM practitioners find kink to be a form of self-healing precisely because it gives them space to explore painful beliefs, memories, and sensations and to recontextualize them in a way that leaves them feeling powerful rather than powerless.

It may seem like a cop-out to end this chapter by saying that what's normal for you is what's normal for you. And yet that is the only honest answer I can provide. The secret here is to understand that what is normal for you is not normal *only* for you, that there are millions of other people who share your experiences with sex and sexuality: people who wonder if they're enough in bed or wish their partner were willing to have sex just a little more often; people who struggle to accept their right to sexual pleasure or even to experience sexual pleasure at all; people who have grown up in a world that has not treated sexuality with the same joy and positivity that it affords every other area of adulthood.

What would it have looked like if we had been as well prepared to make choices about sex and intimacy as we were about college planning and career development? How would it feel if we could discuss our bedroom curiosity and conflicts as naturally as we discuss parenting challenges and housekeeping life hacks? What's normal for you is what's normal for you. And it can be beautiful in whatever form it takes.

MORE TO READ ON THIS TOPIC

Becoming Cliterate: Why Orgasm Equality Matters—and How to Get It

Laurie Mintz

Guide to Getting It On, 10th ed.

Paul Joannides

Sizzling Sex for Life: Everything You Need to Know to Maximize Erotic Pleasure at Any Age

Michael Castleman

7

What Does "Normal"
Kink Look Like?

We now know that an interest in kink is normal and that kinky people are normal people. But one of the most common questions I hear from my clients is "But is *my* kink normal?" Even when we intellectually understand that BDSM is a valid relationship dynamic and that those who practice power-exchange relationships are (throwback to Wednesday Addams!) just like everyone else . . . there's often a secret worry that we might be the outlier—the one truly weird person in the crowd of otherwise totally ordinary kinksters. This worry is born, in my opinion, out of the secrecy that has historically (and necessarily) surrounded the BDSM community.

Like all groups who have traditionally been "underground," BDSM practitioners have long been early adopters of new technology in their efforts to connect with their communities. In the mid-twentieth century, from roughly 1940 to 1980, placing classified ads in various specialty audience magazines (nudist, pulp pinup, detective/adventure, and leather were popular options) and the personals section of the newspaper was a primary strategy for finding one another. Using coded language that only other members of the kink community might recognize, they used the mail to connect with potential dating partners and private-event organizers. Today, social media and the internet have made it incredibly easy to find like-minded communities, although many users have to balance their desire for connection with the potential risk of someone undesirable (a parent or employer, perhaps) finding their online profiles. On one hand, it's wonderful that people can find one another and experience a community that supports and affirms their desires and their relationships. On the other hand, even though information is more accessible, you still have to know where to look to find it.

Today, the most popular BDSM/kink community website is FetLife, which claims to have over 10.5 million users around the world.[1] Intentionally designed to *not* be a dating site, FetLife allows users to post blog entries and photographs, join groups focused on every possible niche fetish and relationship dynamic, advertise or find local events, and more. These events typically fall into one of four overarching categories:

MUNCH/SLOSH: Meetup events held at either a restaurant (munch) or bar (slosh), these are casual social events typically organized around a location and/or kink lifestyle. You may see a TNG (The Next Generation) munch for eighteen- to thirty-five-year-old kinksters living in New York City, for example, or a slosh for Orange County femme-identified submissives. Munches and sloshes are held in public spaces, are not sexual events, and are intended for community networking and friendship formation.

PUBLIC CLASS/WORKSHOP: There are dozens of small nonprofits and individual kink educators around the country who offer short classes on specific skills (such as ichinawa, or slow rope–style bondage), fetishes (safe wax play), or kink lifestyles (pony play for beginners). Some classes are held in private homes. Others rent community spaces such as restaurant or library meeting rooms. Most require a nominal fee, and many occur in conjunction with a munch or slosh. Depending upon the nature of the class, it might be possible that participants would engage in some degree of nudity or physical contact with others, but classes and workshops do not typically include overtly sexual activities.

PLAY PARTY: Play parties are private events organized by individuals or local clubs/groups for the purposes of engaging in BDSM play. Some businesses, such as private dungeon spaces or sex clubs, have a variety of bondage furniture and gear that individual kinksters might not be able to afford for themselves. Play parties give attendees the opportunity to access these resources, meet other like-minded kinksters, and potentially indulge in a BDSM scene (which may or may not include sexual contact, depending on the specific event rules). Attending a play party does not obligate one to participate (many folks love to attend and watch others play, to consensually scratch their voyeuristic itch), and some events offer color-coded wristbands or lanyards that allow attendees to signal their desire for interaction and play (or lack thereof) before even being approached.

CONFERENCE/CAMPOUT: What happens when you combine all of the first three into one glorious multiday event? You get a conference! Or depending on location and time of year, a campout! There are many popular BDSM events hosted each year that bring people together for socialization, classes and workshops, mingling and networking, and yes, even some kinky play, all in one spot. The largest of these events can bring together several hundred attendees of all backgrounds, orientations, and levels of kink engagement. Some of the most well-known events include:

- Beat Me in Saint Louis (St. Louis, MO)

- Beyond Leather (West Palm Beach, FL)

- Camp Crucible (Northern Maryland)

- Dark Odyssey (Baltimore, MD)

- DomCon (Los Angeles, CA, and New Orleans, LA)

- Folsom Street Fair (San Francisco, CA)

- KinkFest (Portland, OR)

- KinkyKollege (Chicago, IL)

- Southwest Leather Con (Phoenix, AZ)

And many more! For those seeking to learn more about or find friendship within specific fetish communities, there are:

FOR ABDLS, LITTLES, AND THEIR CAREGIVERS:

- Chicago Age Play Convention, a.k.a. CAPCon (Chicago, IL)

- TeddyCon (Allentown, PA)

- West Coast Jungle Gym (San Diego, CA)

FOR PET-PLAYERS:

- Equus International Pony Play Event (Los Angeles, CA)

- Ponies on the Delta (New Orleans, LA)

- Puppypalooza (Los Angeles, CA)

FOR ROPE PRACTITIONERS:

- BeachBind (Hedonism II Resort, Negril, Jamaica)

- RopeCraft (Chicago, IL)

- Tethered Together (Stanford, CA)

NEGOTIATIONS

As a general rule, kinksters don't take much for granted. They do not assume that just because both parties are interested in the same thing (for example, a foot-worship scene), that everyone understands what that means and what such an evening would include. They take the time, before clothing comes off, to discuss what each person desires and what they want to avoid. They discuss signals to call things to a rapid halt and ways to know that everyone is having fun. This negotiation practice doesn't just occur for one-off encounters either. Many, if not most, kinksters will insist on negotiating their long-term relationships as well, taking the time to ensure that everyone is on the same page about what commitments are being made, what behaviors are expected, and how conflicts will be addressed. In my premarital work with couples (of all flavors and orientations), I encourage them to emulate the BDSM negotiations model. What does this look like?

As in most things, different kinky people have developed different negotiation techniques. I am a fan of the model taught by Midori, a shibari rope expert, kink author, and American Association of Sexuality Educators, Counselors, and Therapists (AASECT) certified sex educator who teaches negotiation skills to kinky people around the world. She breaks this process down into five phases:

INFORMATION GATHERING: The time to make sure everyone is on the same page regarding their desires for the scene. Asking questions about power exchange and who will take the lead/cede control during the scene. Being curious about each other's cues and how to tell if the moment is going well and being received favorably. How to recognize when something isn't being enjoyed. Inquiring about turn-ons and turnoffs, safety protocols and limits. Determining up front what aftercare is expected when the scene is over.

THINKING AND CREATING: A collaborative conversation about the space you're in (physically and emotionally), the tools and toys you have available, and the kind of mood you'd like to create for one another. Discussing fantasies and ways in which you might be able to act on some of those imaginative desires. Holding space for each person to not only brainstorm their sexual desires but also to share their ideal physical and emotional sensory reactions.

WHAT IF?: Time for each partner to consider all the possibilities that the space and resources might afford and to suggest ideas without fear. Looking not only at the sex toys you have available (vibrators, paddles, etc.) and the ways in which they are "meant" to be used but also at the myriad of non-sexual resources available (clothing, light, water, etc.) and to suggest creative ways to leverage these to enhance the experience of the scene. At the same time, this is an opportunity to set limits without hurting feelings.

REFINEMENT: Once a general understanding has been reached regarding what will happen, what may happen, and what should not happen, taking time to ask specific questions that clarify and refine everyone's vision for the scene (or even relationship) is important. Asking not only "Do you want me to strike your butt with my hand?" but also "Do you want it to feel stingier, like a slap, or more thuddy, like a punch?" Seeking deeper understanding about the prioritization of the ideas and sensations you've discussed thus far is helpful as well: "I know you said you want to feel loved and protected but also overpowered and overwhelmed. Do you want to feel more loved or more overpowered? Do you want less protection at certain times?" Midori advises us to "avoid saying 'Do you like that?' or 'Is that okay?' as they may answer with what they think you want to hear."[2] The negotiations process throughout should feel collaborative and never coercive. Everyone involved should walk away feeling heard, included, and respected. If that is not the case, then BDSM play should not proceed.

NOW WHAT?: Once the fantasies have been shared, the opportunities explored, and the boundaries defined, the final step is deciding the practicalities. When will this scene happen? Where should it happen? What do we need to have on hand? Who will be there? The logistical details are the last part of the negotiations process because they should serve as a container for, and not a constraint on, the scene you have worked together to build.

Negotiation as the foundation of BDSM is crucial to our understanding of mixed vanilla-kink relationships. There is no place within BDSM for ultimatums or coercion.

"This is just who I am, deal with it."

"If you loved me, you would . . ."

"I can't help myself."

These phrases and others like them have no space within consensual kink. Every relationship dynamic, every stand-alone scene, is predicated on open and enthusiastic negotiation that by definition includes discussion of and respect for boundaries. The responsibility for emotional and behavioral self-regulation is on each person, and no BDSM relationship or play should be entered into if one is feeling pressured or unheard. You have the right to ask for what you want, need, and desire. You have the right to be heard and to have those requests respected. You are under no obligation to fulfill the desires of anyone who does not properly negotiate them with you. Without negotiation, mutual agreement, and ongoing renegotiation, it is *not* consensual kink—period. Speaking of which . . .

DOMESTIC DISCIPLINE

Years ago, when I was conducting field research for my first book, *The Leather Couch: Clinical Practice with Kinky Clients*, I attended a weekend-long event for spanking aficionados in Texas. I had been working with gender, sexuality, and relationship minorities for a good long time at this point and was fairly confident that I knew what to expect from the weekend. I was wrong. Many members of this particular community of southern spankophiles did not consider themselves to be part of the BDSM community. One speaker in particular began his demonstrations by warning the audience that this was a wholesome activity undertaken by God-fearing Christian people who care deeply for one another and that anyone who thought that adult bare-bottom spanking was dirty or kinky should get their minds out of the gutter. This was my introduction into the world of Christian Domestic Discipline (CDD).

Within some corners of the conservative world, primarily among self-identified evangelical or traditionalist Protestants, there is a small but thriving community of people who believe that male heads of household have a patriarchal right and responsibility ("dominion") to use corporal punishments to keep their wives on the correct spiritual and marital path. This is a controversial lifestyle that often blurs the boundaries between fetish play and domestic abuse. Consensual kink is predicated on equality of expectation.[3] It is quite possible for consenting adults to mutually negotiate a relationship agreement whereby one partner agrees to act as a 24/7 lifestyle submissive, or slave, with opportunities available to speak their needs and request adjustments to the dynamic. CDD, as implemented by the small number of fringe families who practice it, is *not* BDSM.

Practitioners of CDD teach their daughters and wives that "under God's law, the social class of men are the only ones who have full autonomy. Women are to be under the authority of men in the home, the church, and society at large."[4] In fact, one leading voice within this movement describes the importance of marrying women when they are quite young because they are malleable and grooming them to be model surrendered wives is easier: "From a biblical perspective, grooming when used in the sense of a husband conditioning his wife to be in complete subjection to him and molding her behavior to his preferences is not evil or immoral. But rather, these actions are righteous, holy, and required of husbands by God."[5] Dossie Easton and Janet Hardy, authors and kink educators, share the idea that power exchange is only possible when the person submitting has power to give. Consensual BDSM is predicated on the notion that the submissive partner is making a choice to cede their authority to another person in a way that is mutually agreeable, adjustable, and able to end things if either party finds that it does not serve them.[6] Likewise, I encourage my clients to envision the reverse of whatever power-exchange dynamic might be and to consider if it would be possible. Could there exist a female-head-of-household CDD family? Proponents of this particular relationship dynamic would say no, that such a structure is unnatural and anti-biblical.

When someone says there is only one "right" way to hold power in a relationship, that power structure can only exist in one form, with one person (or gender) holding the control. When one partner lacks agency, having been quite literally groomed to assume a role that they are taught is necessary for their eternal salvation, there cannot be equality of expectation.

FETISH PLAY

At this point, you're already well aware of what a fetish is, but I want to take a moment to acknowledge how we tend to respond to and think about fetish play. Fetishes often show up in pop culture as either the punch line of a joke or as a signal to the audience that a particular character is somehow "off" or unsafe. This is incredibly disheartening because sexual fetishes are actually incredibly ordinary! Numbers range from one in six[7] to one in four[8] people reporting they've explored at least one fetish, while nearly half say they have at least one fetish they're interested in, even if they haven't had the opportunity to act on that interest.[9] Some of the most common fetishes include:

- feet/toes
- voyeurism
- piercings
- hair
- body fluids (such as spit, breast milk, or urine)
- clothing associated with legs/butts, such as stockings and skirts

- footwear/shoes
- underwear
- costumes
- gender or age-play

Many of my clients, both kinky and vanilla, want to understand *why* they have the sexual fetishes that they do. The science of fetishism is not well studied, and like most things related to one's sexual and relational preferences, there is probably not one definitive answer that is "right and true" for all fetishists. The two most popular theories are the signals crossing theory, which is most often used to explain foot fetishes, and the early childhood imprinting theory. The signals crossing theory recognizes that "specific locations in your brain correlate to specific locations on the body. The part of the brain that is triggered when the genitals are stimulated is adjacent to the part of the brain that is mapped to the feet. It is theorized that some people have an overlap in neurons of these areas. Basically, the boundaries of the map overlap, meaning that feet can cause sexual arousal in a person."[10] The signals crossing theory may explain why foot fetishes are so incredibly common (47 percent relative frequency[11]) and that they may stem from, quite literally, how we're wired. Early childhood imprinting theory offers us two possible scenarios for how a fetish might develop. "The conditioning model theorizes that fetishes develop when a stimulus is paired with sexual thoughts or behavior. . . . The trauma model is based on the idea that fetishes are rooted in either emotionally or physically traumatic experiences in childhood or adolescence. This also includes unresolved emotions from childhood or growing up in sexually restrictive households."[12]

Since we've already explored the connections between trauma and kink (reminder: researchers have not found any), I'm inclined toward the conditioning theory. We know that new neural pathways are forming all the time in our brains and that exposure to various stimuli (both sexual and not) can literally alter the way the brain is wired. This is called neuroplasticity and is central to our understanding of behavior. It's important to recognize that understanding how and why a specific behavior develops is *not* the same as pathologizing that behavior or deciding it's bad. Neuroplasticity is also important for how we study in school, for how we learn how to socialize as children, and in make-or-break lifestyle habits such as smoking and exercise. The fact that psychologists want to understand where fetishes come from does not mean that these researchers consider having a fetish to be a bad thing. It just is, and they find it (like so many of the differences we find in people), fascinating.

DAY-TO-DAY DOMINATION

Thanks to pop culture, when most people think of living a BDSM lifestyle, they picture a leather-clad dominatrix living in a Victorian mansion or high-rise penthouse, where the red-painted walls are lined with a variety of devious-looking racks and other torture devices and a shirtless man in a collar waits on them hand and foot. More often, BDSM life looks like a sub-urban schoolteacher and her accountant husband creating and maintaining a set of small, personalized rules and rituals that they enact for each other in between making breakfast and driving car pool, going to church and volunteering for the local Rotary Club. Day-to-day D/s looks (in the words of Wednesday Addams) "just like everyone else." A day in the life of a D/s couple might look something akin to the following:

Helene wakes up at 7:00 am when her alarm goes off. She slips out of bed, dresses quietly, and goes downstairs to make breakfast for the family. Once the scrambled eggs are just about done, she brings a cup of coffee upstairs to Sage, who is still sleeping. She closes the bedroom door, kneels by Sage's side of the bed, and gently squeezes their arm to wake them up. Sage smiles, gives her a kiss on the forehead, and takes the coffee. When their cup is empty, Sage takes a heavy silver necklace, Helene's day collar, off of their nightstand and clasps it around her neck. They go downstairs together to have breakfast with the kids before the bus comes. Sage and Helene each fill their plates, as well as the kids' plates, and they sit at the table together. Helene watches and waits until Sage has picked up their fork and taken their first bite before she begins to eat. After breakfast, they hug the children, and Helene loads the dishwasher before they both head to work. On her lunch hour, Helene steps into the washroom and stands in front of the mirror. She recites the affirmation that Sage has prescribed to her ("I am calm and confident. I am loved and I am owned.") before sending them a quick text to let them know that she has completed this task.

After work, Sage picks up the children and takes them to their scout meeting, where they are a scoutmaster. Helene texts Sage to let them know that she is leaving work and to ask if they have any requests for her before she returns home. Sage instructs her to drive halfway home, find a secluded place to park, and to masturbate under her skirt—stopping before she orgasms. She is to take a photo of her wet fingers after completing this task, then to continue on with her commute home. Upon returning home, it is Sage's night to cook dinner. Helene helps the kids with their homework. When they sit down to dine, Helene once again waits until Sage has taken their first bite before picking up her fork. They put the children to bed together and then spend some time together, watching television. Sage sits on the couch while Helene sits on the floor in front of them. Sage brushes Helene's hair while they talk about the events of the day. Just before bed, Sage goes into Helene's lingerie drawer and selects the bra and panties they want her to wear the next day. They go to bed around 10:00 pm. Helene and Sage have sex and Sage tells Helene that, because she did such a good job with her masturbation assignment that afternoon, they will allow her to orgasm tonight. Delighted and expended, they fall asleep in each other's arms.

Daily D/s

(My husband and I) have a monogamous 24/7 D/s dynamic. I am the submissive and he is the dominant. I'd describe us as having a very loving, fulfilling, and healthy relationship. We are very happy, affectionate, and communicate well. I'd say we have one of the happiest relationships of everyone in our orbit. However, it's a long story full of infidelity, misunderstanding, fear, assumptions, and perceptions.

We've been together around thirteen years, and for much of that we were monogamous in theory. He cheated several times, which severely damaged our relationship. We had a lot of discussions about what he'd been looking for when he cheated—a submissive rope bunny—and how I craved the freedom—from my demanding, very visible, and high-powered job—that came from having a Dom. After so many years together, it was like a veil had lifted and we perfectly understood each other. He paid attention to all the things I'd asked him for or enjoyed over the years and shook his head and said, "A blind man could have seen it. I just didn't see you."

Our days look much like they did before we started our dynamic. Very few people know it exists, and many of the things that changed aren't necessarily unusual or visible. Each day I have a series of tasks to complete, starting with doing affirmations in the mirror and texting him that they're done. I have to do this by 10:00 am every day. Many of the other things are related to my own care: I have to drink a specific amount of water, eat two actual meals each day, exercise at least three times a week, etc. He chooses my panties for the day before he goes to sleep; when he wakes up, I've gotten his work uniforms ready for him, and I make the bed as soon as possible after he gets up. He cooks dinner each night and does the grocery shopping and washes and dries all the clothes; I fold and put away the clothes and handle finances and family logistics like appointments and car registration. When one of us is very busy or sick or whatever, the other picks up the slack. He brings me water every night before bed; on nights he works, he gets it and puts it on my nightstand before he leaves. I have to wear my hair a certain way once a week, and wear a dress at least once a week, and he brings me flowers at least once a week. I also have to keep regular bikini wax appointments and shave my legs twice a week. We have a calendar checklist app to keep track of daily and weekly tasks. I'm not allowed to open doors when we're out together, aside from obvious things like the bathroom door. I must walk on his left side unless that side is closest to the road with no barrier between. These have created some comical "debates" and situations, like, can I press the button to call the elevator? Technically it's what opens the elevator door—lol. This simply looks like chivalry to most people.

As far as most people can see, our relationship looks like any other happy vanilla marriage, but our dynamic is always there; it's an ingrained part of our relationship. There are the realities of work and kids and responsibilities to manage that need to happen as equals, and it's helpful for us to maintain lines of communication that lets each of us know when something is a family/partnership discussion versus him as my Dom giving me an instruction or me as his sub making a request. There's little inside flashes, things like me ordering coffee after 7 (which is against our rules), which might result in him subtly rubbing the leather cuff I gave him (inscribed with a code that translates to "Yes sir") and giving me a meaningful look, or I might reach for a door without thinking and hear him loudly clearing his throat (to correct me).

In my regular life, I have a big personality and am in charge of damn near everything, and I am very confident and don't require a lot of praise. As his submissive, doing things specifically to make him happy, that's very different. A dynamic changes little things like that, that you don't realize until you're in the moment, and if your partner doesn't communicate those things and they continue, it can fester and really cause a lot of emotional damage.

One of the challenges was for him to realize how much it affected me for him to do little things, like not responding back to my text that my affirmations were done or acknowledging and praising me for completing all my tasks. A good dynamic is a much deeper bond than even a marriage. When you are giving up your autonomy to someone else, or when you're accepting responsibility for another person, there's an incredible amount of trust that goes into that. He was often not a good husband. He's a much better Dom, and it has made him a better husband. He notices my moods more, picks up on my facial expressions or tones of voice in a way he never did before, because as my Dom he's responsible for me and my happiness and safety. As his submissive, I actively look for ways to help him or make him happy, or I do little things to defer to him that I never did before.

Everything that we do is intertwined. We communicate so much better. We're more open and honest, much more affectionate, and much more in love than we ever have been. Every day we take time to hug, really embrace, and share a quiet moment of content together. And the sex is mind-blowing! Having that amazing trust and openness and knowing you can say anything, ask for anything, try anything, and your partner will not judge you for it is so freeing. I don't have to hold in my emotions or hold back, and he can finally talk about sex and his desires without embarrassment or fear that I'll be disgusted and leave him. More than once I've mused to myself that BDSM saved my marriage. We could never go back to being vanilla or even bedroom-only. In our dynamic, we've found everything we ever wanted and so much more than we ever dreamed possible. I would not recommend entering a dynamic to save a relationship. Yes, I believe it saved mine, but that's because it was what was missing. It was what we both always wanted.

—Noel, 38

PLAY PARTNERS

In the BDSM community, the play partner is a relationship dynamic that serves a delightfully utilitarian purpose: facilitating a scene that may not otherwise be possible, for any number of reasons. Play partners are often friends (sometimes close, sometimes casually) who occasionally engage in BDSM play with each other. Scenes with a play partner may occur because one or both players are single or at an event alone and wouldn't otherwise have someone to engage in BDSM with. Alternately, play partners can help to fill a skill gap in an existing relationship. For example, a husband in a monogamous D/s relationship might encourage his wife to seek out a play partner who is skilled in Florentine-style flogging, because she wants to have that sensory experience and he lacks skill in that area. Some play partners have long-standing relationships where they engage in various BDSM activities without romantic expectations or a power-exchange dynamic that extends beyond the length of the scene. Many play partnerships are platonic, focusing exclusively on BDSM play without sexual intercourse or emotionally intimate contact. Some play partnerships fall under the umbrella of "pickup play" where two people who might not otherwise know each other connect long enough to negotiate a specific scene, then go their separate ways. In many of the mixed-desire relationships that I've worked with, play partners can be a wonderful option to help fill the desire gap between romantic partners. A vanilla spouse might tell their wife that while they have no interest in BDSM play at all, they're comfortable with their wife seeking out platonic friendships with people who *are* kink-identified and who can help meet that need for her without threatening the emotional/romantic relationship between spouses.

LEATHER FAMILIES

The idea of a chosen family has become fairly mainstream over the last twenty or so years. We encourage our children to call our closest friends "Auntie" and "Uncle" without demanding genetic ties. We form blended families through divorce and remarriage. We form families without any religious or legal documents at all. Family is who we choose to keep close, and we take for granted that these choices will be accepted and affirmed without question. For the LGBTQIA+ community, however, the idea of chosen family is born out of centuries of social isolation and familial rejection that is ongoing and very, very real. While LGBTQIA+ youth make up only 7 percent of the youth population, 40 percent of homeless youth are LGBTQIA+. Half of all LGBTQIA+ young people experience a negative reaction from their parents when they come out, and more than 25 percent are kicked out when they come out.[13] Because so much of kink culture developed through and with the queer community, and because so many kinky people have experienced similar rejections and stigmas—both institutional and deeply personal—the leather family has been one way that (often, but not exclusively) queer kinksters have created chosen families for themselves.

In the 1940s and '50s, many gay men returned home after World War II and either experienced this same rejection by their families *or* chose not to share their identities at all and simply decided to remain near the cities they were discharged at following their service (primarily in New York and San Francisco). They found one another within military-influenced clubs, opened by their returning peers, and quickly formed what we now call "leather bars." This community today is known as the Old Guard leather community: a highly structured (now sexually integrated) community of BDSM practitioners who carry on the traditions developed by these members of the "greatest generation." One of the traditions that has come out of this world is the idea of the leather family. For those who have seen the phenomenal show *Pose* about 1980's ball culture, imagine close-knit friend groups that become chosen families . . . but wearing more black leather than sequins.

Leather families are those that have bonded through the leather lifestyle and have elected to join together as a family. A leather family generally has structure and protocols in place as well as rituals. The only way to become part of the family is by invitation. Each family is different. . . . It is strictly a Master/slave association with respect to all members of the family.[14]

On many kink-centric social media sites, you will see titles such as "sister/brother of," "under the consideration for," or "household member with," used to indicate these chosen family ties. Leather families offer education for those who are drawn toward the Old Guard culture, who crave close ties with people who "get" them and their desires, and (for many still today) the same practical and tangible support that a family provides—housing, cooperation, assistance, affirmation, and care. Membership within a leather family is an unusual and special opportunity that expects deference and dedication but is not typically a sexual or romantic bond.

Houses

Some leather families join together to form a common household, with multiple members of the chosen family cohabitating together. Most do not. Separate from the world of Old Guard leather, there are occasions in which one dominant and multiple submissive partners all live together (or who spend a majority of their time together) under the same roof. A BDSM household is typically headed by the dominant. There may be a senior or "first" submissive who takes on a right-hand role to the dominant, overseeing day-to-day household operations and acting as a leader of the other submissives while remaining deferential to the dominant head of household. Unlike leather families, the relationships in a BDSM house are typically sexual and polyamorous. In some houses, the submissives have emotional/sexual relationships with one another as well as with their Dom. Others might be mono/poly, where the Dom has sexual relationships with each of their submissives, while the subs are sexually faithful to the dominant alone. BDSM houses are not common; however, they would be considered a "normal" relationship model within the kink community. The opportunity to join a BDSM house (particularly when one's partner is not interested in taking a dominant role in the primary relationship) can be one strategy for meeting the desire difference between kinky and vanilla partners, particularly when they are already polyamorous or open to the notion of an ethically nonmonogamous relationship.

There are many ways that kinky people have found to build relationships and community around them in a world that has shamed and stigmatized them for centuries. Intentional relationships, both romantic and platonic, with others who understand you is a primal human need. Safety, a sense of belonging, and the knowledge that we matter are core elements of Maslow's hierarchy of needs. It is incredibly difficult to become self-actualized human beings in the absence of a supportive, affirming community.[15] For many kinky people, this supportive, affirming community exists in their household or online. Others are fortunate enough to live in areas that afford them opportunities for socialization—such as munches, sloshes, and conferences—with others who "get" them and their relationships. This deep understanding, the connection that occurs without explanation because they share a common language ("munches") or culture (leather, collars, etc.) can make it so much easier to form the kind of romantic relationships we desire as well, particularly when those too fall outside of the mainstream.

MORE TO READ ON THIS TOPIC

Hearts and Collars: Twenty Years in a Power Exchange Relationship

Dan and Dawn Williams

The New Topping Book and *The New Bottoming Book*

Janet Hardy and Dossie Easton

Playing Well with Others: Your Field Guide to Discovering, Exploring, and Navigating the Kink, Leather, and BDSM Communities

Lee Harrington and Mollena Williams

8

When One Flavor Isn't Enough

If you are like many of my clients, you might be feeling a little skeptical about how your vanilla and kinky desires can work together—especially after I've mentioned the idea of folks having some form of kinky contact with a person who is not their committed partner. The notion of a play partnership or joining a leather family or D/s house can feel like scary propositions for people who have been in traditionally monogamous relationships. Your hesitation makes perfect sense. The idea that BDSM and kink can exist separately from emotional and romantic connection, or even sexual contact, can be difficult for those of us raised in Western mono-normative cultures. Yet the idea that monogamy *is* the norm is much more of an ideal than an actual social reality. In America, approximately 4 to 5 percent of the population identifies as polyamorous,[1] while an estimated 20 to 30 percent (depending on sexual orientation) of the population states that they've engaged in some form of consensual nonmonogamy.[2] These are the numbers for folks practicing *ethical* nonmonogamy! We've already discussed the rates of unethical infidelity that occur in seemingly committed relationships. In other words, monogamy is an ideal that many of us say (or think) we want . . . but one that can be incredibly difficult to maintain across a life span. Perhaps this is why there is such a vast spectrum of ethically nonmonogamous relationship styles to choose from today.

Before we proceed further, I want to reassure you that this chapter is *still* focused on answering the question "What does normal look like?" The following section is intended to describe what normal can look like in a nonmonogamous relationship, keeping in mind that there is a difference between what is *normal* and what is *normative*. As sociologist Nicki Lisa Cole puts it,

"Normal" refers to that which conforms to norms, so while norms are the rules that guide our behavior, normal is the act of abiding by them. "Normative," however, refers to what we perceive as normal, or what we think should be normal, regardless of whether it actually is.[3]

Whole libraries have been written about the structures and practices of ethical nonmonogamy, and this brief chapter is not the place to try to reinvent that wheel, nor are the descriptions that follow an attempt to convince you that polyamory is the right "prescription" to cure your relationship challenges. As with any sexual practice or relationship model, it won't work for everyone, and that's okay! But for some of you, especially those who are already drawn toward other nonnormative relationship dynamics, some version of ethical nonmonogamy may be a valid path forward. The tricky thing is that because ethical nonmonogamy is not often portrayed in popular media (When was the last time you saw a sitcom about an open marriage?), many of the people who might be drawn to these relationship styles aren't aware that they are a viable option already practiced by many of their friends and neighbors. Let's look at what these can look like for folks in mixed kinky-vanilla relationships.

POLYAMOROUS PARTNERSHIPS

Our culture is pretty clear about what constitutes a "normal" adult relationship: You fall in love with someone (*one* someone!), you have sex with them, you decide you want to have them in your life all of the time, and you make a mutual agreement to do so. That dyad (group of two) forms our normative understanding of what it means to have a long-term relationship. For many people, however, the idea of only sharing their life (and their bed) with one person feels incredibly stifling. They want romantic love, emotional connection, sexual desire, and deep commitment, and they want to experience these with multiple people simultaneously. This can take many forms. Sometimes the two partners form romantic relationships with other people, either on their own without including their "dyad" partner (parallel poly) or by forming friendships with their partner's other partners (their metamours) and facilitating opportunities for their "dyad" partner to do the same (kitchen table/backyard BBQ poly). Alternatively, some people don't separate "my" partners from "your" partners and instead choose relationships where three or more partners each make an equal romantic and emotional commitment to the others. Regardless of who is romantically connected to whom, these variously shaped groups of partnerships and metamours are referred to within the community as "polycules"—a play on molecules and the many chemical bonds they form. The BDSM houses we discussed earlier constitute one form of polycule.

There are dozens, if not hundreds, of ways in which people practicing ethical nonmonogamy build long-term, committed relationships without the assumption that those commitments become less valid if more than two people are involved. One of the foundational understandings in polyamory is the notion that it can be unreasonable to expect one person to be your everything: your friend, your lover, your fellow hobby enthusiast, your sports-team cheering section, your horror-movie film-fest date, your coparent, your roommate . . . much less your owner, your house boi, your kitten, your bootblack, or your master. Those who identify as poly and kinky may find it easier to get the latter needs met when they aren't reliant on the hope that their only partner's erotic desires will align with their own. Instead, they have the space and the support necessary to form loving, committed BDSM relationships with partners who desire that as well, while their vanilla partner relaxes at home with a soft blanket, a good book, and the warmth of compersion.

Kitchen-Table Poly

I am currently partnered with Josh; we have been dating for about nine months, although Josh first called me his girlfriend about five months ago. I mostly date men, however, I do have sexual attraction toward women as well (which varies day to day and depending on how drunk I am; the more I drink, the more "lesbian Sabrina" comes out). For me, the queer label is one that is as much political as it sexual. It identifies that I'm not "straight" without having to explain the complexities of my sexual and romantic attraction. It does not assume that I am in a monogamous relationship, nor that I am vanilla. For me, all of these aspects (attraction toward men and women, in a polyamorous relationship, and submissive/ BDSM/kink identified) are an important part of who I am. Queer encompasses all of that.

I would describe my relationship with Josh specifically as one that is based on mutual support, a deep sense of caring for the other person, and one that feels incredibly safe and secure. As someone with a background of religious trauma in childhood, as well as other types of trauma, this sense of safety is incredibly important to me. Early on in our relationship, I told my therapist "my nervous system feels safe with him." It's a hard feeling to describe, but I don't feel on edge like I normally do. I feel like I can relax and be myself.

I have met all of Josh's partners and his partners' partners. Josh lives with one of his partners (Emilie), and her other partner (Jake) is over on Saturdays, which is when Josh and I spend the day together. If I am visiting him at his house, it's not uncommon for all four of us (plus whatever gaggle of children happen to be present that day!) to sit down around the kitchen table, have dinner together, and enjoy talking. While I don't have any other partners at the moment (although I am dating), should I develop another relationship, I'd welcome Josh meeting them, as would he. For me, it feels comforting knowing the other people involved in Josh's life and Josh (eventually) knowing mine. It helps me feel a greater sense of community and connection.

I didn't necessarily create this dynamic as much as I fell into it. I am equally as happy in polyamorous relationships as I am in monogamous relationships. Navigating a mono-normative culture is definitely a big challenge. It's hard to explain to your coworkers that you spent Thanksgiving with your boyfriend, his wife, her boyfriend, your boyfriend's other girlfriend, her other boyfriend, and her other boyfriend's wife. It's also hard to explain to your family. I have a map of our polycule that I made for situations like these that I tend to hand out. It's definitely hard to know how open I can be at work. My family tries to be supportive, but I often experience microaggressions.

I enjoy the sense of community that kitchen-table polyamory brings. While I don't have a super-close relationship with my metamours and their partners, I know that if I were to need something, especially urgently, they would be there to help me. I also enjoy the ability to seek out relationship needs in other partners. I believe that our culture's focus on one partner being able to meet all of your relationship needs is incredibly toxic and completely unsustainable and unrealistic. The ability to say to a partner "Okay, I need this thing and you can't/are not able to provide it and I'd like to search for it elsewhere" is such a rewarding experience. It allows for open communication about what is and isn't working in a relationship and means that I can stay in a relationship with someone and still get my needs met.

—Sabrina, 38

FRIENDS WITH BENEFITS

For those of us who might not want a(nother) long-term relationship but who still want the opportunity for safe and enjoyable sexual pleasure, there exists the "friend with benefits." A friend with benefits (FWB) is similar to a kinky play partner: someone safe that you are friendly with and are attracted to enough to want to sleep with (or scene with, in the case of play partners) but who doesn't hold the same emotional place in your life that a boy/girlfriend or other partner might. They are, in essence, your booty call. The perfect person to invite over for a beer, board game, and bedroom Friday night, but not someone you'd necessarily introduce to your grandma. For some kinky people, the terms *play partner* and *FWB* are used interchangeably. Others draw a distinction between relationships with BDSM but no sex (the former) and those that include some form of sexual/genital contact (the latter). For some folks in mixed vanilla-kink relationships, it's a lovely compromise to have an FWB who shares their fetish and who offers a trusted outlet to explore desire without feeling like a threat to the primary partner. I have worked with many couples who consider themselves monogamous but create space in their relationship agreement for the kinkier partner to have an FWB who enjoys the types of play the primary vanilla partner would rather skip. This is definitely a relationship model that must be carefully negotiated and transparently maintained, but it can work well for committed couples who find themselves at an erotic impasse.

HOOKUPS AND MONOGAMISHNESS

The term *monogamish* was coined by Dan Savage to describe his own relationship with his husband, in which they were romantically committed to each other but allowed to have casual sex with other people. While the idea of sexual pleasure being disconnected from emotional betrayal has long been a touchstone of the polyam/ethical nonmonogamy (ENM) community, many couples who consider themselves "monogamish" would not necessarily use the terms *polyam* or *ENM* to describe their relationship. One of my favorite client couples was a pair who both traveled extensively for work. They described their relationship dynamic as "monogamous in Michigan." Monogamish couples are honest about their extramarital activities. Some couples negotiate elaborate logistical and behavioral ground rules for what choices, partners, and behaviors are allowed during these encounters. Like BDSM, some folks may request some form of debriefing and processing from their partners afterward. This transparency is what differentiates monogamishness from infidelity. In fact, the transparency is an added benefit for many who find it incredibly erotic to hear about their partner's sexual encounters after they occur.

One step removed from monogamishness is the hookup. Hookups are casual sexual encounters that occur between people with no expectation that the relationship will continue once the clothes go back on. Often hookup partners are found through apps such as Tinder, Grindr, Feeld, and the like, as well as websites such as Adult Friend Finder and some other mainstream dating websites. What differentiates monogamishness from hooking up is often a matter of degrees. While (ideally) the ground rules for both monogamishness and permission to hook up are prenegotiated before anyone steps outside of the committed dyad, couples who create space for hookups often have a "Don't ask, don't tell" policy in place when they return home. They are more than happy to give their partner room to roam, but they are happiest when the details are left at the door. This can be an acceptable arrangement for folks in mixed kinky-vanilla relationships since ethical nonmonogamy can feel like a "kinky" practice in and of itself—the idea that they can openly and honestly negotiate an agreement for the kinkier partner to have their needs met without the pressure to participate (or even hear the details about it) at all. Relationship structures that provide less communication require more trust from those involved. These arrangements can be a workable solution when the relationship is otherwise strong, but I highly recommend that any couple considering exploring monogamishness work with an ENM and kink-affirming certified sex therapist to help form their initial relationship agreements and navigate potential conflicts until you find your footing.

SWINGING

You might have noticed a common theme in the ENM dynamics we've discussed so far: they tend to be relationships or experiences that people have individually, away from their other partner(s). In a kitchen-table poly relationship, you and your whole polycule might gather for a cuddle-pile viewing party of the latest superhero blockbuster, but it's unlikely that everyone is going to wind up in bed together after the credits roll. If you practice parallel poly or monogamishness, you might never meet your metamours at all. I have worked with many people who understand their partner's erotic differences and who want to encourage them to explore and experience everything they desire but who want to remain an active presence and participant in the sexual activities their partner pursues. Many of these couples find a home within the lifestyle otherwise known as swinging.

> *Swinging has been referred to as the group closest to traditional coupledom among those who are non-monogamous, due to the way in which couples typically portray themselves publicly as heteronormative and monogamous. The commitment to the partner remains the main focus and—when threatened— often results in the couple forming rules to protect the primary relationship (e.g. keeping certain forms of sex sacred to the couple). The removal of secrecy and dishonesty is attributed to the continuation of this group; couples are able to engage in fantasies together, resulting in an increased trust and openness in the relationship.[4]*

In other words, swinging is ethical nonmonogamy that puts the dyad relationship first and that happens together. Swinging might include threesomes or group sex or could involve the primary partners having sex with others in the same general proximity (same bed, same room) to each other. Sometimes swinging takes the form of one partner watching the other have sex with someone else and enjoying the scene. Mixed kinky-vanilla couples may find attending lifestyle events such as play parties or adults-only resorts to be an intriguing way to explore the potential for kink in their own relationship. It's one thing to listen to your partner describe their love for wax play, for example. It's quite another to watch your spouse writhe under the dripping candles of someone who prides themselves on their sexy sadistic skills. Seeing your partner engage in BDSM with others can open us up to the idea of bringing those same activities into the bedroom at home and experiencing the thrill of being the one to bring them pleasure. Even if we walk away still uninterested in participating in BDSM or fetish play ourselves, we've still created space for our partner to have the experiences they desire openly, honestly, and with the person they love most at their side.

RELATIONSHIP ANARCHY

The term *relationship anarchy* (RA) was coined in 2006 by Andie Nordgren, an Icelandic political anarchist who wrote a short manifesto describing a relationship model that did not have hierarchies, rejected most relationship rules and expectations (including sexual fidelity), and that sought to prioritize the needs, wants, and desires of the people involved rather than adapting to social norms and traditions. According to Nordgren's manifesto, the key elements of relationship anarchy are:

- Love is abundant, and every relationship is unique.

- Love and respect instead of entitlement.

- Find your core set of relationship values.

- Heterosexism is rampant and out there, but don't let fear lead you.

- Build for the lovely unexpected.

- Fake it 'til you make it.

- Trust is better.

- Change through commitment.

- Customize your commitments.[5]

As one RA practitioner put it, "I want relationships based around consent and communication, I believe I can love as many people as I choose, I value each relationship I have independent of the others, sex doesn't necessarily come into play regarding who my important people are. I highly value autonomy and direct communication, and therefore I won't ask you for permission to do things, but I will talk to you about how you feel for as long as you need to!"[6]

This emphasis on agency and autonomy (without hierarchy or permission-seeking) that relationship anarchy affords can feel intimidating or liberating, depending upon your perspective. Folks who are uncomfortable with traditional notions of marriage or the ways in which Western society prioritizes romantic love over other emotional bonds, who want the freedom to express love and affection in multiple ways toward multiple people without being asked to label or rank their relationships, should consider learning more about this radical free-love philosophy.

Relationship Anarchy

Over the last almost fifteen years, I've been many varieties of nonmonogamous. At nineteen I met a nice guy I wanted to date who asked what I knew about polyamory and open relationships (nothing, and, well, I'd heard of them; I read Dan Savage's column) while he was asking me out. I would say the rest is history, but it was actually a pretty complicated process of self-discovery and feeling out boundaries over my next several relationships (some of which overlapped, because I didn't go back to monogamy in a formal way ever again).

I've been romantically partnered with Ken for six years. We don't live together. He lives a few towns over with his other two romantic partners (of eight and fifteen years) and their children. I have shared custody of my kids (ages five and eight) with my ex-partner and ex-metamour; the kids are at my house fifteen days a month and at my coparents' home the other half of the time. I also have two play partners, ages thirty-two and thirty-six. We met in 2016 and, honestly, I was expecting our relationship to be a short-term play partnership. But one of the advantages of both being nonhierarchical is that we could adjust as our feelings moved beyond the scope of our initial plans. Over the years that followed, there have been lots of fluctuations in my situation—from two romantic relationships to one to two again to one again; a platonic dating situation turned into a regular ongoing kink play partnership (composed of mostly rope and knife play) with my best friend between our regular hangouts; and post-pandemic I've made a new kink-and-sex-based play relationship with a friend from the local kink scene.

I've been able to rely on an underlying sense of knowing myself and my values and boundaries when making new relationships. An RA outlook on my relationships gives me the freedom to build the relationships I want, how I want them at the moment, and change them when they don't serve me and my partners. Honestly, the transitions from other forms of polyamory to a nonhierarchical/flexible RA-based approach have mostly been challenging because it can be perceived as a "downgrade" in your existing enmeshed relationships; and being sensitive to feelings about that while still being honest about wants and needs is important. Figuring out which of your expectations and wants are yours and not just "scripts" that are socially determined can be really freeing but *super* hard.

I see one of my play partners about once a month for a kinky play session alone, and another approximately once a month with friends at social things (and talk most days—we're best friends); and the other sporadically—we'll not see each other for a few months and then weekly for a month and then "wander away" as we get busy. Adult friendship is complicated, and adding play didn't suddenly make any of us more reliable. People who are willing to do the work of having ongoing conversations about personal boundaries and to base relationship agreements on those and keep them relatively fluid are generally people who are willing to build meaningful connections, whether they be of long or short duration. The long ones are flexible enough to be functionally forever, even if they aren't forever romantic or forever sexual. It's given me scope to accept that the romantic and D/s relationships in my life don't have to also be my coparenting relationships or my financially entangled relationships to be among the most meaningful ones I will have and to be people who will matter to me even when some aspect of our relationship changes. Consider the many relationships you have with someone. If you live with a romantic and sexual partner, you're their lover and their roommate and maybe also a collaborator on parenting or finances. You can always negotiate stepping back only some. Embrace the joys in *today,* and if your structures and agreements no longer contain any joy and gratitude today, recognize what parts of your connection did and renegotiate to emphasize those. It's better to make challenging transitions and release things than to stew in pain "because we might make it work." Always negotiate.

—Laura, 33

RADICAL MONOGAMY

Some of the relationship models we've discussed here might feel just as scary, or scarier, than the notion of BDSM itself. I've worked with many clients who worry that bringing elements of kink into their relationship is a slippery slope toward a nonmonogamous lifestyle they have zero interest in. The good news for these people is that while there is a happy Venn diagram of folks who are both kinky *and* nonmonogamous, there is no expectation that one requires the other. There are thousands of happily vanilla people in polyamorous relationships. Likewise, there are many, *many* monogamous kinksters. Welcome to the world of radical monogamy.

Too often we form monogamous relationships not because it's what's best for ourselves and our lives but because we believe that we *should* be monogamous, because our religion says so, because we're heterosexual, because it's what our relatives do, because it's what our cultural group expects, because we have children, or because it's the only option we've been taught. Radical monogamy says that monogamy doesn't have to be a reactive choice; that we have the agency to consider a wide variety of relationship models and to choose the one that is best suited to our nature and our relationship—including a closed dyad.

Radical monogamy holds space for queer relationships, kinky relationships, non-cohabiting relationships, for all kinds of relationships that feel countercultural or subversive and yet still desire an exclusive sexual and romantic commitment. Radical monogamy agrees with the nonmonogamous voices who point out that it can be difficult for one person to be all things for their partner and encourages healthy independence and deep friendships with others. Radical monogamy is a proactive choice that is not superior to other choices but simply the right one for those involved.

Jericho Vincent, the Jewish essayist and speaker, put it best when they said,

I've always wanted a gigantic love. I wanted to be one person's joy and delight and I wanted them to be mine. . . . Then I grew up and I was told that was ridiculous, unrealistic, and unhealthy, so I gave up on monogamy and practised polyamory. But now I've come around to believing that all those other people's messages were wrong. If approached with intentionality, effort, and a willingness to grow, it is possible to have a love that's big and magical. . . . Some people really do want monogamy; I think that's a healthy desire and I hope that for those who want it, radical monogamy will offer a totally new portal to a joyful, healthy, magical kind of love.[7]

MORE TO READ ON THIS TOPIC

The Heart of Dominance: A Guide to Practicing Consensual Dominance

Anton Fulmen

PolySecure: Attachment, Trauma, and Consensual Nonmonogamy

Jessica Fern

Sex Outside the Lines: Authentic Sexuality in a Sexually Dysfunctional Culture

Chris Donaghue

9

When It All Feels Hopeless

Some of the readers holding this book in their hands right now picked it up because they were afraid that their relationship could not survive the challenges facing it. And that fear is valid—not because the challenge of a mixed vanilla-kinky relationship is particularly difficult compared to other relationship issues but because the outcome of divorce is incredibly common in our culture. Today, roughly half of American marriages will end in divorce. This number grows to 60 percent of second marriages and nearly three-quarters of third marriages. Couples who marry at older ages or who practice a religious faith are less likely to divorce than their younger, more secular peers,[1] although this may vary based on religious identity because some faith groups are more accepting of divorce than others. Judaism and Islam have religious divorce rituals, for example, while the Catholic Church prohibits its members from divorcing.[2] There are no statistics that speak specifically to how kink-vanilla relationship tension affects a decision to divorce, but researchers have found that infidelity, lack of commitment/compatibility, and conflict are frequently cited as reasons why couples decide to separate.[3] It's easy to imagine how a couple deciding to end their mixed vanilla-kinky marriage might use one of those categories to describe their situation. Let's talk a little bit about what to do when you just . . . can't.

HONORING WHERE YOU ARE

Remember that negative feedback loop we discussed back in chapter 3? I want to be very clear—this is a picture of pain:

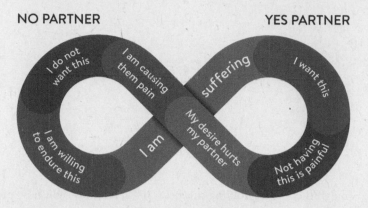

NO PARTNER   **YES PARTNER**

I do not want this

I am causing them pain

suffering

I want this

I am willing to endure this

I am

My desire hurts my partner

Not having this is painful

EMOTIONAL FEEDBACK LOOP

And I want you to know that it's okay, at any stage, to acknowledge that it's become too much to bear, to understand that it is *always* okay to opt out of suffering. You do not have to feel like you are causing your partner pain by asking for too much or denying their desire. You don't have to feel selfish or greedy, frigid or sinful, for wanting or not wanting whatever it is your soul craves. The Jewish tradition teaches that marriage is too sacred, too holy, to defile by staying in a bad one, and that we honor the sanctity of this bond by refusing to let it become something that torments us. Or as Elizabeth Gilbert puts it, "The only thing more unthinkable than leaving was staying; the only thing more impossible than staying was leaving. I didn't want to destroy anything or anybody. I just wanted to slip quietly out the back door."[4] The life coach D. Ivan Young takes this notion of ending without causing harm a step further and asks us to imagine the harm our decision will mitigate: "If anything, you're correcting a mistake that was hurting four people, you and the person you're with, not to mention the two people who you were destined to meet."[5]

READ THIS IF YOU'RE VANILLA

There is nothing wrong with being a vanilla person who wants to have a vanilla relationship with your partner. You are not being a bad partner. You are not being demanding. You are not being unfair. You certainly aren't broken. Sexual connection and compatibility is the single most important factor we must take into account when considering long-term relationships, because it involves the most intimate parts of our bodies, hearts, and minds.

You have every right to the relationship you want most, and you are under no obligation to qualify or compromise on that if doing so would cause you long-term pain or discomfort. You are allowed to ask your partner for anything and everything you need to be happy, safe, and content in the relationship . . .

. . . and no is always a valid answer.

You can ask your partner for anything, but you cannot control their behavior. You cannot make demands or issue ultimatums that coerce them into giving you the vanilla life of your dreams. Here's what you get to control:

You decide what you're willing to tolerate.

You can ask your partner to set aside BDSM or whatever their fetish might be and to live a vanilla life together with you. And they get to say yes or no. You don't get to influence their answer . . . but you get to respond to it. Your locus of control lies in what you're willing to tolerate in your relationship and in your life. If they decline your request, that's their choice. And no is sacred. You then get to decide whether you're willing to tolerate a relationship that includes a kinky partner or if that's a deal breaker for you. Either option is a valid choice, but that's where your power lies—not in forcing your partner to give you what you need but in deciding for yourself if their answer is one you can live with. Neither path is necessarily easy, but one might be the better path for you. And that's okay.

READ THIS IF YOU'RE KINKY

There is nothing wrong with being a kinky person who wants to have a kinky relationship with your partner. You are not being a bad partner. You are not being demanding. You are not being unfair. You certainly aren't broken. Sexual connection and compatibility is the single most important factor we must take into account when considering long-term relationships, because it involves the most intimate parts of our bodies, hearts, and minds. You have every right to the relationship you want most, and you are under no obligation to qualify or compromise on that if doing so would cause you long-term pain or discomfort. You are allowed to ask your partner for anything and everything you need to be happy, safe, and content in the relationship . . .

. . . and no is always a valid answer.

You can ask your partner for anything, but you cannot control their behavior. You cannot make demands or issue ultimatums that coerce them into giving you the kinky life of your dreams. Here's what you get to control:

You decide what you're willing to tolerate.

You can ask your partner to consider exploring BDSM or whatever your fetish might be and to live a kinky life together with you, or at the very least to give you space to explore your kinks alongside them. And they get to say yes or no. You don't get to influence their answer . . . but you get to respond to it. Your locus of control lies in what you're willing to tolerate in your relationship and in your life. If they decline your request, that's their choice. And no is sacred. You then get to decide whether you're willing to tolerate a relationship that puts limits on your kink expression or if that's a deal breaker for you. Either option is a valid choice, but that's where your power lies: not in forcing your partner to give you what you need but in deciding for yourself if their answer is one you can live with. Neither path is necessarily easy, but one might be the better path for you. And that's okay.

EXPERIENCING GRIEF AND LOSS

In her seminal 1969 book *On Death and Dying*, psychiatrist Elisabeth Kübler-Ross developed a five-stage adjustment pattern to describe the process she witnessed in people who were processing the death of a loved one. Since that time, her model has been used to explain how humans grapple with losses ranging from the death of a child to the loss of a job. Her work has been used to guide change management in businesses and to help families trying to cope with a loved one's drug addiction. One time in life when we often experience this process is when dealing with the evolution or end of a marriage. Here I want to explore these stages as they relate to the conversations my clients have with themselves and with each other about their original hopes and expectations for the relationship versus where they find themselves once they realize they are misaligned in their responses to kink.

DENIAL: This is the stage that first brings many of my clients to see me. They sit across from me and say things like, "This isn't really who they are.

It's a trend, a phase" or "I can wait. I know their reaction when I told them was suboptimal, but if I just keep quiet and wait, they'll change their minds." They come to therapy in the desperate hope that if *they* do the work, their partner will change. Don't get me wrong, change is possible in many, if not most, relationships. When we genuinely love our partner and desire their happiness, we are often willing to adapt to and explore new things that would never have occurred to us on our own. But when the disclosures have occurred, the learning has happened, and the boundaries are defined? When they've done everything "right" and their partner still is not the person they wish that they were? This is when my clients often begin to exhibit what Stark has called "relentless hope." Relentless hope is "a defense to which the patient clings in order not to have to feel the pain of her disappointment in the object, the hope a defense ultimately against grieving. The patient's refusal to deal with the pain of her grief about the object . . . fuels the relentlessness with which she pursues it, the relentlessness of her hope that she might yet be able to make the object over into what she would want it to be."[6] At this point in the grieving process, particularly when other aspects of the relationship are quite positive, this denial of the reality of who their partner is and what they desire (or not) can keep both partners clinging to the relationship long past the point when they've reached an intimate impasse.

ANGER: For kinky people, one of the scariest points in the separation process is here, when the anger rises. This might be the vanilla partner's anger at realizing that their partner's fetish is not going to magically disappear if they just wait long enough. It may be the kinky partner's anger at having a genuine need or a core aspect of their identity rejected by someone they love deeply. Sometimes this anger is played out in ways that can be deeply damaging to the individuals involved. BDSM practitioners have a long history of being denied child custody or visitation due to stigma associated with their private relationship practices.[7] Thankfully this trend is changing as the mainstream community becomes more familiar with what BDSM is and is not. However, it is sadly not uncommon for kinky people going through a divorce to have their private thoughts, feelings, and experiences weaponized against them by a spouse grappling with their own anger and lashing out. My goal as a clinician is always to help divorcing partners separate as gently and kindly as possible.

To that end, one kink-affirming divorce attorney recommends the following steps to protect both spouse's intimate lives and identities from being weaponized during this stage of the grieving process. These are good habits for parents to maintain regardless of their relationship status; they model a healthy understanding of safe, sane, and consensual kink practices and can serve to mitigate risk if you do ultimately decide to walk away:

To protect themselves as much as possible, parents should take the following steps:

- Keep all bedroom activities in a locked bedroom and out of earshot of all children.

- Keep all sex toys, equipment, erotica (including tasteful art), or other sexually explicit material in a locked drawer and away from children.

- Take care that children are not exposed to a BDSM dynamic outside of the bedroom.

- Password-protect your computer. If children have access to your computer, use a separate (password-protected) user account for any lifestyle-related online activities.[8]

BARGAINING: When a mixed vanilla-kinky relationship begins to fail, bargaining can look a lot like negotiation. The difference is that negotiation comes from a place of individual power (and discussions of how best to share it), while the bargaining of grief is usually experienced as a desperate effort to head off circumstances we feel powerless to prevent. Many of my kinky clients offer to swear off any form of BDSM or fetish play forever. The idea of losing the relationship is so painful that, in the moment, they genuinely believe that they can sublimate their desires (sometimes including individual practices such as masturbation, solo play, or viewing erotic content) indefinitely. Needless to say, this is not only unlikely but also unfair. For vanilla partners, the bargaining may take the form of pushing (or even violating) their own boundaries in a desperate effort to be "enough" to satisfy their kinky partner. We've spent a great deal of time together exploring setting and expanding boundaries. But when vanilla people allow their boundaries to be violated as a part of their grieving process, this can quickly turn dangerous for everyone involved. Boundary violations that we do not speak or that we allow in the hopes that they will result in a different outcome (restoration of the relationship, partner happiness, our own pleasure) are often experienced as trauma. These experiences, while consensual in the moment, can cause harm that we may end up blaming the kinky partner for "inflicting" after the fact. It is critical to our own mental health and to the process of gentle separation that both partners recognize when boundary creep or the offering and accepting of boundary violations occurs in our attempts to bargain away our grief. During this time, more than ever, it is crucial to remind ourselves that *no* is sacred.

DEPRESSION: When relationships end due to desire discrepancies or differences in orientation, we go through a period of mourning the life we thought we were going to have. This experience is a common aspect of separations, even when the relationship ends for reasons unrelated to intimacy. We naturally mourn the lives we thought we were going to have. Even when we avoid separation and choose to compromise, that process still requires us to let go of the idea of what our relationship was going to be in favor of what it is becoming. It makes sense that this can lead to depression. We all carry a vision (often from childhood) of what our ideal relationship and family life will look like, and anytime that vision is altered, we must mourn and adjust. However when change occurs because of a crucial difference in the needs or mindsets of the partners, it can be hard not to internalize that as a statement on who we are. "If they loved me more, they'd have been willing to try harder," or "I wasn't worth fighting for," or "They loved <insert difference here> more than they loved me." These thoughts turn the issue from a mismatched relationship to an inadequate person (ourselves) and can result in feelings of depression on top of the grief we're already working to process. The most important thing you can do right now is to remember that you are not your relationship and that a relationship's end (or evolution) is not a statement on the people involved. You both can be (and likely are) wonderful people and worthy partners deserving of love . . . and still just not fit together.

ACCEPTANCE: Whether our relationship ends or evolves, the final form it takes is usually one that is a much better fit for our needs and our lives. Separation or divorce creates the opportunity for us to build a new relationship with someone whose sexual and relational needs better match our own. Renegotiation and redefining the existing relationship gives us the chance to build a partnership where everyone can be their most authentic self without fear, subterfuge, or judgment. How can we look at either of these outcomes and not see them as improvements over where we started? At the end of the day, no matter how difficult this process is, I promise you will come out the other side happier and more whole. Or, as the journalist and humorist Helen Rowland put it, "When two people decide to get a divorce, it isn't a sign that they 'don't understand' one another, but a sign that they have, at last, begun to."

YOU DESERVE TO BE HAPPY

You deserve to be happy. Full stop. No one will ever get me to agree that someone deserves to be miserable or must sacrifice their own joy in order to be a "good" parent or partner. In fact, by prioritizing our own sense of contentment, we're better able to be present and engaged for those who rely on us. That's why flight attendants tell everyone to put on their own oxygen masks before assisting others—if we are denying ourselves what we need, we can't possibly be effective in meeting the needs of anyone else. This is not to say that we'll be happy at every moment and in every experience. Each one of us will absolutely have times that are hard, painful, tragic, and unfair. We cannot always control what situation we find ourselves in. But we can choose how we respond to them.

The end of a relationship can be a painful experience, but it does not have to be a damaging one. This process begins when we recognize the emotions that serve us and those that steal our joy. "Anger is not power—it's weakness. Expressions of anger drain your reserves. While holding on to anger can be compelling and might even seem morally or ethically important, anger is antithetical to peace."[9] When we recognize our anger, our hurt, our grief, and choose to respond to these feelings as the emotional wounds that they are, we can tend to them as we would a physical injury—with gentleness, compassion, and kindness. We decide what we're willing to tolerate (from others and from ourselves). When we make a conscious effort to prioritize grace and kindness in how we navigate this transition, we are choosing happiness—for ourselves, for the person we have been in relationship with, and for any children we might have. Endings are almost always hard. But they don't have to be harmful.

As I've said, I tell each of my clients that they are my client, not their relationship. And I encourage them to choose happiness for themselves as often as possible. This means choosing not to pursue revenge or position themselves as martyrs. This means fostering safety for themselves and their children through their decision-making and behaviors. This means asking themselves, "Which action will require less emotional energy?" and opting to de-escalate their responses as an act of self-preservation rather than niceness toward others. It means choosing kindness not because our partners deserve it, but because *we* do. We may desperately want to remain in a relationship that is ending with or without our consent. We might be the one making a wrenching decision to walk away in order to live a more authentic, connected life. We can't always control the situation we find ourselves in, but we can choose how we respond to it. The Buddhist teacher Pema Chödrön wrote that "we can make ourselves miserable, or we can make ourselves strong. The amount of effort is the same." You decide what you're willing to tolerate. You are not obligated to tolerate misery simply because you are in the midst of transition. Choose happiness, even when it feels like the harder choice.

BUT WHAT ABOUT THE KIDS?

Most every parent is aware of the impact that divorce can have on children. The negative consequences of marital "failure" have been hammered home ever since no-fault divorce became legally accessible in the United States. In 1969, California (under the leadership of then-Governor Ronald Reagan) became the first state to allow spouses to request divorce without citing a specific cause. New York was the last state to allow no-fault divorce in 2010. Prior to the passage of these laws, married people could only end their relationships if they met very specific legal requirements such as abandonment, infidelity, or cruelty. Persons seeking a divorce had to file a claim in court and show evidence to prove that their situation met the criteria for these conditions. Otherwise, the expectation was simply that people would stay together and endure, which is not a solution that makes marital conflict magically disappear.[10] This is important to note because while we tend to emphasize

the impact that divorce has on children, the toll of a high-conflict parental relationship can be just as high. The research shows that "both parental
divorce *and* growing up in a high-conflict two-parent family appear to be
linked with long-term detriments in children's psychological adjustment."[11]

The ideal, of course, is a happy and harmonious family. Unfortunately we
can't always be ideal. When a separation becomes inevitable, it's important to
know that the kids can be okay. There's been very little research conducted
into the *benefits* that divorce can have for children, but what is there offers a
bit of hope. Social scientists are beginning to find that many of the negative
outcomes associated with divorce may have been due, at least in part, to social
stigma around divorce in the 1980s and '90s when most of these studies were
conducted. As one research team put it, "Children of divorced parents typically respond to the cultural meanings of divorce."[12] In other words, the kids
were affected most by being treated by teachers and relatives, classmates and
coworkers like the sad products of a broken home. That stigmatizing reaction
that we might today refer to as "concern trolling" is what caused the most
harm. Shifts in cultural norms over the last twenty years have dramatically
increased our understanding and acceptance of diverse personalities, lifestyles, and family structures. These shifting cultural messages may very well
impact future studies of childhood outcomes related to divorce.[13] For now, we
can take comfort in the findings of researchers who have been interviewing
college students about the impact their parents' divorces have had on them.
Some of the benefits these young people reported include:

- greater feelings of empowerment, in terms of independent goal
  setting and decision-making[14]

- "increased sense of responsibility, maturity, self-confidence, and
  inner-strength"[15]

- heightened relationship savviness and an appreciation of the work
  and skills necessary to sustain a healthy relationship[16]

- deeper empathy toward others and perspective taking, including
  a "higher acceptance of their parents' choices, weaknesses, and
  strengths"[17]

- more tolerant of people with different viewpoints[18]
- "exposure to different family values, tradition, and lifestyles"[19]
- greater sense of awe and gratitude[20]

There is an adage commonly used by therapists who work with children and families and those who work with couples: it's not about the quantity of time you spend together; it's the quality of that time. For spouses and for children, marriages are healthiest when they are happiest. When it is possible to be happy together, I believe we should make every effort to support that goal. If there comes a day when you realize that the quality of the relationship doesn't justify the toll it's taking on you or your children? I believe that we should make every effort to facilitate a separation that is grace-filled, compassionate, and kind. Children do best when they have positive relationships with their parents, regardless of where those parents live. We protect our children when we honor our partners, even as we move toward a day when they no longer hold that role in our lives.

Divorce

(My husband) was working from home and was wearing a T-shirt that had a little tab on it just like a baby would wear, where you hook the pacifier on a little string so it doesn't get lost. I could not understand why a grown man would wear a shirt like that. Another time he kept texting me at work that he wanted to go to the doctor because he was feeling sick. He finally went, and he said he was ultimately diagnosed with a kidney infection. He came home with the biggest diaper I've ever seen in my life—and he's not a big guy, either! But it was like a diaper with plastic pants connected to it all in one. He would sometimes walk around in nothing but that diaper. It was so unattractive to me, but I knew he had a kidney infection and so I just dealt with it. I walked into the bathroom when he was standing in nothing but that diaper and I finally asked him, "How long is this kidney infection going to go on?" He responded, "Okay, I won't wear it any-more." Somewhere deep inside, that's when I realized that he was wearing it by choice.

I know now that he is an ABDL (adult baby/diaper lover) and I see it as part of his identity and something as much a part of him as anything. Once I realized it was a thing for him, I told him to take one of the spare rooms and turn it into "his" room. In my mind, I thought that this way, he could be him-self in his own space and still be the person I married in our common areas. But my acceptance made it grow like ivy, and his fetish began to take over. He took that spare room and turned it into a literal nursery with a twin-bed-sized crib. He made his own clothes that were exact replicas of children's clothing, such as having snaps down the inside seams of the pants. He made himself onesies from old shirts. He made baby food. It began to overtake everything. He struggled negotiating bound-aries, but so did I. I showed my best friend his little nursery room, because I knew that if I didn't show someone, they just couldn't understand it. And she stood there, looking around in awe—like she was standing in a museum. And she said, "If someone didn't see this, they would never understand it, the extent to what you're going through." And I wasn't trying to shame him; I just needed someone to validate me.

I made the decision to divorce when the clinical sexologist we were working with was working on my identity development. I finally realized that my husband was gay and he had a fetish, and while that was fine for him, it was doing nothing for me and I was again sacrificing my sexual health and happiness. His fetish/kink played a huge role in my decision to leave. I knew that I was causing him harm because I was so very turned off by his kink, but at the same time I also realized that I deserved to be happy and have a fulfilling life, with a man who desired me. I finally decided it was time to take that step and I initiated divorce.

It was strange. We slept in the same bed literally until the day I moved out of our home. My relationship with my ex is amicable, but we really only text on very rare occasions. We are both supportive of each other's ways of moving forward in life. I am now in a monogamous relationship of three years. Neither of us are really interested in kink or BDSM. We are pretty vanilla and we're content.

I would encourage you to try to understand that this may be a very big part of their identity that started at a very young age and plays a very important role in their life. For most people, trying to make it go away just brings pain and anxiety. Negotiate. Ask yourself what you *can* do to include the fetish. Seek a qualified sex therapist. At the same time, don't sacrifice your own happiness for someone else.

—Holly, 51

MORE TO READ ON THIS TOPIC

Better Apart: The Radically Positive Way to Separate

Gabrielle Hartley and Elena Brower

Love Yourself Like Your Life Depends On It

Kamal Ravikant

The New "I Do": Reshaping Marriage for Skeptics, Realists, and Rebels

Susan Pease Gadoua and Vicki Larson

10

Cocreating the Future You Want for Yourself (and Each Other)

I n 1967, psychologists Thomas Holmes and Richard Rahe created a scale designed to measure the impact of stressful or traumatic life events on an individual and to use this measure to predict the person's susceptibility to chronic, stress-related health problems.[1] Holmes and Rahe identified forty-three specific stressful life events and assigned them each a weighted value (referred to as "life-change units") based on how traumatic these events were perceived to be by the participants in their study.[2] They found that folks with a score of 150 or less experienced low stress and generally good health. The middle group scoring 150 to 299 were described as experiencing moderate stress, which Holmes and Rahe found represented a 50 percent chance of being diagnosed with a chronic health condition related to stress. Those who scored 300 or more life-change units were enduring significant stress and were 80 percent likely to experience chronic health problems. Since it was first introduced, the Social Readjustment Rating Scale (or SRRS) has been proven to be a highly reliable measure of both present stress and future health.[3] Why does this matter to us today? Among the forty-three stressful events identified by Thomas and Rahe, getting married within the last twelve months holds a value of 50 life-change units, while a marital reconciliation after a challenge comes in at 45, and sex difficulties ranks high on the list (#13 out of 43) with a score of 39 life-change units. This means that for many readers of this book, their overall stress score is starting out anywhere from 39 to 89 before we even consider other significant life events![4] I tell you this because I think it's important to understand: the distress you experience as a result of navigating sexual differences and challenges is real, valid, and worthy of your attention. The impact of these feelings is not less-than because they are sexual or kinky in nature. Sexual stress is still *real* stress. But there's good news!

REMEMBER "GGG"?

In chapter 3 we touched on Dan Savage's mantra of "good, giving, and game." It turns out there's a lot of research that supports this idea! The concept of partner responsiveness, or "the extent to which a person feels that their partner is aware and supportive of their needs," is one of the cornerstones of relationship science.[5] The impact that having and being a responsive partner has on a relationship cannot be understated. Partner responsiveness is connected to how we perceive and handle stress, affect, intimacy, trust, affirmation, communication, sexual desire, and sexual satisfaction.[6] The more we feel like our partner understands and is responding to our needs, the happier we are as people and the stronger the relationship will be.

Responsiveness means different things to different people, so let's be clear about what we mean when we talk about partner responsiveness in the context of mixed vanilla-kink relationships. The way that a vanilla partner responds to their kinky partner's disclosures has the potential to build a foundation of strength for the evolving relationship. "Research has shown that both sexual and nonsexual self-disclosure lead to greater sexual satisfaction . . . and that mutual self-disclosure results in greater relationship satisfaction, leading to greater sexual satisfaction."[7] The very process of having the conversations you've likely been having as you navigate your differences has created opportunities for deeper happiness both as individuals and as a couple. For kinky people, being able to talk about and share your desires with your partner, even if they don't act on them with you, builds closeness and reinforces the relationship bond.[8] For vanilla people, you don't *have* to share or act on your kinky partner's desires in order to be responsive to them and reap the benefits that your responsiveness creates. Everyday acts of kindness toward each other—nonsexual touch, loving words, and helpful actions—have been shown to increase our sense of relationship closeness.[9] This might look like watching a movie that features BDSM themes or buying your partner a new fetish object to enjoy privately. It might mean a gentle touch or a kind gesture from the kinky partner toward their vanilla love. It might look like incorporating words and terms that help them feel seen and accepted. It may take the form of creating simple rules or rituals with your partner that can honor that aspect of themselves without crossing the fences you've defined.

If you can find common ground to act on the fantasies, the benefits become even clearer: "Individuals who make more frequent changes in their sexual habits to accommodate a partner, such as changes to sexual frequency or type of sexual activity, have partners who report greater relationship satisfaction."[10] I know what you're thinking: "What's in it for me?" Research also tells us that, with a few exceptions, our partner's sexual satisfaction is connected to our own sense of relationship satisfaction![11] In other words, when we make an effort to please our partner, we both end up happier for the effort.

SEDUCTION VERSUS NEGOTIATION

Many clients I've worked with over the years dislike the idea of negotiating their relationship agreements. Vanilla folks particularly, who don't have the same cultural connection to the negotiations process that kinksters do, tell me that it feels too businesslike and unsexy. They're not interested in role-playing as corporate attorneys nitpicking the minute details of a contract. They want to be seduced, which makes perfect sense to me! When negotiation is done well (Midori's model we discussed earlier being the prime example!), it should feel like seduction. Not a seduction in the way that pickup artists (PUA) and other would-be Casanovas use the term, where one person uses flattery, negativity, and deception to persuade another to submit; but rather seduction as a way to foster desire for closeness, or what ethicist Sarah LaChance Adams calls "ethical seduction." Unlike the PUA's efforts to wheedle someone into agreeing to a specific outcome (typically no-strings-attached hookup sex), ethical seduction "is propelled by the desire for proximity but to an unforeseen end. And this uncertainty is the key to its benefits. If one presupposes the goal of seduction, that its outcome should be a date, sex, or marriage, then the other person becomes either the object of, or an obstacle to, one's plans."[12] BDSM negotiations and ethical seduction share this commitment to mutual participation and openness to possibility. Adams describes ethical seduction as including several key elements that are also found within the process of negotiating a scene or relationship dynamic:

- centering the person being seduced as an "active and creative participant, there to co-determine the ultimate purpose of the relationship"[13]

- awareness of the seducer's power (socially, relationally, etc.) and judicious restraint in their sharing of knowledge

- awareness of and respect for each partner's identity, as well as an understanding that these are not static traits but can and will change over time

- curiosity about the other person's perspective

- vulnerability in sharing your own worldview and sense of self

- respect for each person's agency and autonomy

- mutual support for each other's independence and appreciation for how our lives and selves interconnect and support each other

- genuine engagement with each other and curiosity (rather than defensiveness) about your areas of difference

- optimism for the future

For many vanilla partners, the negotiation process can feel like an ultimatum if not handled delicately. Because the goal of negotiation is to find some common ground, it by necessity assumes that the end result will be some degree of BDSM engagement, which can leave some vanilla folks feeling coerced. Using the language of ethical seduction and weaving the negotiation conversation into a greater framework of playful self-disclosure and mutual appreciation can help mitigate this and foster a space where positive experiences are possible for both partners. These conversations can be scary. They require a degree of trust and vulnerability that some of us might not want to undertake, and yet the very acts of having these conversations and experimenting with the ideas that come up as a result have known benefits for our relationships. "Relationship satisfaction is higher when partners engage in shared novel and challenging activities. Such activities allow for increased closeness, as partners learn about themselves and each other through these activities."[14] Being willing to engage in ethical seduction and negotiation opens us up to greater closeness and happier relationships, even when we are challenged to expand our comfort zone or to let go of some of the things we once thought we had to have.

CREATING INTENTIONAL RELATIONSHIPS

I love having these kinds of conversations with my clients. Navigating discovery, processing the feelings that the disclosures bring up, and doing the hard work of choosing love, affirmation, and commitment makes for one of the most transformative experiences the partners I work with will likely experience in their lives. The possibilities that open up for them—the opportunity to redefine what their relationship looks like moving forward in a way that is intentional, collaborative, trust-filled, and hopeful—is an incredible blessing that I feel honored to facilitate. One of my favorite things to witness is the way that partners grow throughout their work together, becoming stronger not only as a couple but as individuals as well. Watching them moving through hurt, confusion, and pain toward a place of strength, confidence, and choice is an amazing thing to see, and this growth is an inevitable part of the healing process. As Chris Donaghue puts it, "Healthy adults do not partake in limiting and self-deprecating inherited belief systems. They critically analyze beliefs and institutions they engage in and create boundaries that meet their own chosen goals. This is a powerful moment when you literally throw away the rulebooks."[15]

Intentionality is the heartbeat of a relationship. Intentional words. Intentional behaviors. Intentional moments. Intentional responses. When we stop reacting to our partners—stop following relationship scripts written by religious, cultural, or family influences that do not serve us—we begin to foster a sense of deep accountability that lets us flourish. Accountability to ourselves, a commitment to bringing our full authentic selves to every interaction with our partners; and accountability to them as well, to upholding the commitments we make and the agreements that we form. To act with transparency and integrity in the relationship. To give them the gift of our truth.

Donaghue says, "Censorship is a symptom of anxiety." When we self-censor, holding back our desires and our fears, we are living in a place of fear that our authentic self will not be loved the way we desire to be loved, that our partner will look at us and recoil. The exercises we have undertaken together throughout this book have given you the tools you need to engage in self-reflection, in transparent disclosure, and in ethical seduction. When we undertake this work intentionally together with our partner, maintaining a sense of authenticity for ourselves and curiosity toward the other, what we create can be truly amazing.

Compassionate Kink

I have a lot of friends in the kink and poly worlds. Kink/polyam/gaming are communities that tend to go together. I'm more than happy to dive into that with a partner, if that's what they enjoy.

Today, my wife's kinks don't really overlap with our sexual relationship. I understand my partner's kinks to be focused on dominance, power exchange, and breath play. I am supportive of her need/want/desire to explore her kinks. She first got involved in doing rope, which led to power exchange, impact play, breath play; she's done a lot of topping scenes with other men, including co-topping men with her female friend. She goes to kink camps and enjoys setting up scenes there.

I tend to have feelings around her being in any sort of submissive position with anyone other than me or in a situation where I am not involved. I think that's due to a lot of cultural norms: "That's my wife." I've been cheated on a couple times in the past, so I have to grapple with those feelings and thoughts at times and separate her out from my past experiences and be more objective about what she's doing, asking me to do, etc. I think her being in a submissive position does bring up some insecurities for me, culturally around "my position" versus that being just an interest that she has that has nothing to do with our relationship. It is not always sexual for her.

BDSM and kink do not play a huge role in our life currently. It definitely wasn't easy. There were times when it was really hard. BDSM and kink were introduced almost immediately prior to a poor introduction to polyamory, so the two were linked in my head and heart for a bit. My wife did some sexual things, pegging, anal play—things that she was performing on (a submissive). There was never penetrative sex for her, but it was a lot to wrap my head around. It felt like cheating because we didn't talk about it first. It felt bad. If we'd been more up front first, I still would have had my struggles, but we could have talked about some guidelines and expectations, and we could have eased into it better. As time went on, I tried to understand where my partner was and where we were heading, and I researched a lot about kink and poly, trying to figure out what these offered her and what they could offer me.

My wife continues to go to kink events, and I have encouraged her. She can indulge her interests. She can exercise dominance and power-exchange desires at these events. I have some minor insecurities that I am able to handle by just keeping myself busy while she is away. We have conversations around desires and comfort levels before she goes to these events. Open dialogue is welcomed and encouraged. I let her practice some techniques and knots on me. Nothing too involved, though. It was not my thing but that is not important.

Be honest with yourself going in and look at those hard questions: How does their involvement with kink . . . impact me negatively? Is it really the big problem that I built it up to be in my mind at first, or is it something I don't need to be stressing about? Talk about everything. Read a lot. Ask a lot of questions, and be okay with the answers. Some of them might be hard to hear, but don't go with your initial reaction. Be willing to take it all in, think about it, and have a conversation, even if it's hard. Do try to expand your comfort zones, even go to events with them. It's one thing to know something, but being there is a whole other thing—just to expose yourself to new things. You might realize there are things you want to explore. Be open to understanding your partner and where the possibilities lie for you.

Do I need this? Not really. But does this open up opportunities for me too, that I might not have thought about before? Yes. It can if you're willing to do the work. This is my life partner, and these are the things that she's into, and so I did as much as I could to understand and support her. I have a pretty happy life right now.

—Dale, 54

THE POWER OF YES

When you first learned about the differences between your sexual desires and your partner's, both of you were likely holding onto many *no's*:

- *No*, I don't want to talk about this.

- *No*, that's not my thing.

- *No*, I couldn't possibly . . .

- *No*, I don't find that sexy.

- *No*, I can't share that piece of myself.

- *No*, I can't understand . . .

- *No*, I'm not going to listen.

- *No*, that's not who I am.

- *No*, they wouldn't love me.

Hopefully, since then you've found some yeses along the way: things that you want, things that you're curious about, things that you're open to exploring, things you feel safe to share. I tell my clients all the time that *No* is sacred.

Yes is also powerful. *Yes* unlocks doors and minds. *Yes* turns toward and not away. *Yes* builds trust, intimacy, and hope. *Yes* is where honesty grows. That's why most wedding vows request an affirmative statement, to look each other in the eyes and say "I do." Renowned sex therapist Tammy Nelson writes, "A one-time promise . . . doesn't cover all of the changes you will go through in a shared lifetime—all the stressors, the arguments, the illnesses, the children, the financial troubles, and the difficulties are part of the natural ups and downs of a relationship. To weather these changes, you need something more. You need an everyday vow."[16] In the context of a BDSM dynamic, these everyday vows can look like the protocols, rules, and daily rituals that affirm and reinforce the relationship agreement. Many vanilla couples have similar unspoken or unrecognized habits that serve the same purpose: a monthly date night, a Saturday-morning coffee routine, a practice of greeting each other with a kiss at the door. These small everyday yeses are the foundation of a strong relationship.

Thoughts follow behavior. When we undertake to make small behavioral changes, our brains cannot help but follow. When we develop this routine of small daily yeses, the everyday vows of intentionality and affirmation, we are better able to consider the larger yes moments that may feel a bit more complicated for us. A willingness, for example, to choose our partner's tie or panties each morning, as a subtle gesture of affection (or perhaps dominance), costs us very little in terms of emotional energy and time spent but can have a tremendous impact on their understanding of our responsiveness to their needs. Yes builds upon yes. And each yes brings us closer.

- *Yes*, I'm okay with you exploring that alone.

- *Yes*, I am willing to refrain from . . .

- *Yes*, I'm okay with you visiting that website.

- *Yes*, we can watch that video together.

- *Yes*, we can use those words.

- *Yes*, I am willing to try to . . .

- *Yes*, we can go to . . .

- *Yes*, you can stay home while I . . .

- *Yes*, I can experiment with . . .

- *Yes*, I am willing to respect that boundary.

No is sacred because it protects the sanctity of our self. *Yes* is powerful because it contains and defines our relationship to others. *Yes* is a promise we make every day. It's a promise that can change shape, certainly. But the commitment to finding our capacity for yes and offering it to our partner is the ribbon that binds our hearts together.

The following chart details a wide scope of what kinky play can look like. For some folks, these activities are sexual. For some, they're pleasurable and sensory but not erotic experiences. Still other people use these activities to shape and maintain their relationships. They do not, in and of themselves, define what kind of relationship the people engaged have to each other. After so much learning, self-reflection, and shared dialogue, I'd like to close this book by doing one more exercise. Talk to your partner about your interest in the activities on the list and what it would look like to include them in your intimate life together. Then use the chart to define your yeses, such as they are today. This could be anything from "Yes, I will do this with you" to "Yes, I'm okay with you exploring that with someone else" to "Yes, I'm willing to learn more before I decide." *Yes* doesn't have to be an action verb. We aren't always committing to do the thing or to do it forever. We may be agreeing to learning more about the thing, to trying the thing once, or to being okay with the thing happening far away from us. That's okay. By creating a space where you both can play safely (together or apart), you are also creating a relationship that is affirming, transparent, loving, growing, and evolving side by side, hand in hand. You can download and print this worksheet at stefanigoerlich.com/with-sprinkles-on-top-worksheets.html#/.

Finding Your Sprinkles Discovery Worksheet

	I Am Curious About This for Myself	I Would Be Willing to Let You Do This To/For Me	I Would Be Willing to Do This To/For You	This Might Be Okay to Do With Someone Else	I Want to Learn More Before I Decide	This Is Outside of My Fence for Now
Bondage						
Blindfolds						
Bondage Furniture (Stocks, Crosses, etc.)						
Bondage Under Clothing						
Bondage/Surgical Tape						
Cages						
Chains						
Handcuffs						
Harnesses (Leather or Rope)						
Hoods						
Immobilization						
Saran Wrap						
Spreader Bars						
Straightjacket						
Tied to Bed/Chair						
Tied Up With Ropes						
Wearing a Collar						
Wearing a Gag in Mouth						
Wearing a Leash						
Wearing Leather or Metal (Wrist/Ankle) Cuffs						
Other:						

	I Am Curious About This for Myself	I Would Be Willing to Let You Do This To/For Me	I Would Be Willing to Do This To/For You	This Might Be Okay to Do With Someone Else	I Want to Learn More Before I Decide	This Is Outside of My Fence for Now
Discipline						
Bathing/Toileting/ Hygiene Rituals						
Chastity/Abstinence						
Choosing Clothing/ Undergarments						
Daily Rituals						
Daily Tasks						
Eye Contact Restrictions						
Household Chores/Cleaning						
Loss of Privileges (TV, Video Games, etc.)						
Ordering/Choosing Food						
Postures/Poses						
Rules/Rule Following						
Speech Restrictions						
Standing/Sitting/ Kneeling in Corner						
Writing Lines						
Other:						
Dominance & Submission						
Age Play						
Begging						
Cigar/Ashtray Service						
Commands/Orders/ Instructions						

	I Am Curious About This for Myself	I Would Be Willing to Let You Do This To/For Me	I Would Be Willing to Do This To/For You	This Might Be Okay to Do With Someone Else	I Want to Learn More Before I Decide	This Is Outside of My Fence for Now
Forced Orgasms						
Kneeling/Bowing						
Name-Calling						
Orgasm Denial						
Ownership						
Pet-Play						
Shaving						
Spitting						
Tea/Coffee Service						
Teasing/Name-Calling						
Using Honorifics/Diminutives						
Wearing a Symbol of Ownership						
Other:						
Sensory Play						
Biting						
Choking/Breath Play						
Clamps or Clothespins						
Hair Pulling						
Hair Brushing						
Ice						
Melted Wax						
Pinching						

	I Am Curious About This for Myself	I Would Be Willing to Let You Do This To/For Me	I Would Be Willing to Do This To/For You	This Might Be Okay to Do With Someone Else	I Want to Learn More Before I Decide	This Is Outside of My Fence for Now
Rough Surfaces (sandpaper, burlap)						
Scratching						
Spiked (Wartenberg) Wheel						
Tickling						
Wearing a Blindfold						
Zapping/Electric Play (fly swatters, prods, wands)						
Other:						
Impact Play						
Belt Spanking						
Face Slapping						
Giving/Getting Bruises or Marks						
Hand Spanking						
Hitting with a Cane						
Hitting with a Flogger						
Paddling						
Riding Crop						
Whipping						
Other:						
Fetish Play						
Boots						

	I Am Curious About This for Myself	I Would Be Willing to Let You Do This To/For Me	I Would Be Willing to Do This To/For You	This Might Be Okay to Do With Someone Else	I Want to Learn More Before I Decide	This Is Outside of My Fence for Now
Corsets						
Costumes						
Feet						
Foreplay/Sex Outdoors						
Foreplay/Sex While Others Watch						
Fur						
High Heels						
Latex						
Leather						
Masks						
Nudity						
Pantyhose/Stockings/Socks						
Sexy Clothing/ Lingerie in Private						
Sexy Clothing/ Lingerie in Public						
Uniforms						
Other:						

PARTING THOUGHTS

Every time I teach a class, whether for certified sex therapists or college undergraduates taking Intro to Human Sexuality, I get the same question: "Isn't it kind of insulting to call people vanilla?" And my answer, every time, is a resounding *no*. The term *vanilla* isn't describing someone who is lacking. It's the rich and beautiful base upon which all other sexual expression is built. To see this most clearly, we only need to look at how actual vanilla is made:

Take the seed pod of a plant grown in lush, verdant, tropical places like Madagascar or Tahiti and split it in half. From there, it is immersed in a neutral base alcohol such as vodka. Within a matter of days, the vanilla bean starts to change the base liquid into a deep amber color. It infuses its scent and flavor into every molecule. And in time, the vodka (which functions essentially as alcoholic water) is completely transformed into a product so rich and delectable that only a few drops is needed to completely transform everything it touches.[17]

"Vanilla" is not the absence of flavor; it is the essence of it. Returning to our earlier lesson about boundaries, vanilla is the edifice upon which we build our fences. One simply cannot exist without the other.

While it's true that pickup play exists and some kinky people engage in BDSM scenes with people they don't have longer-term relationships with, the vast majority of kink is played out within committed relationships. Sure, it can be fun to tie your partner to a rack and flog them with a cat-o'-nine-tails. That can be a hot fantasy, and it feels good for many folks in real life too. But most kink doesn't happen in a dungeon. It happens in the carpool lane and the Thanksgiving dinner, at the doctor's office and in the bedroom. A subtle nod before speaking. A rush to hold the door. A hand on the back of the neck while chatting with friends. A slap on the butt as you pass through the kitchen. These are minute actions that carry powerful meaning—not because of what they are but because of what they say to and about the partners who have created them. Sure, kink can look like head-to-toe latex and some intimidating-looking sex toys. But sometimes kink looks like one partner making dinner while the other is sprawled out on the living room floor with a coloring book and a sippy cup of wine.

The vanilla people that I work with tell me that they want relationships built on mutual love, respect, understanding, gentleness, and trust. Funnily enough, the kinky people I work with also tell me they want relationships that center on love, respect, understanding, and trust . . . Some of them just find the "gentleness" aspect to be negotiable. When we are able to find elements of BDSM that feel good and safe for us, even if we don't label them as "kinky" for ourselves, we are able to create something unique and wholly ours with our partner. It doesn't have to be everything. Maybe in reading this book you discovered that having your movement restricted with ropes or scarves is a sensation you enjoy. The creative constraints of limited motion can certainly enhance the otherwise routine sexual experience! Maybe you learned that it's powerfully effective to adopt a certain stricter tone with your partner and use their full name when you're upset about something: "Michael, you've been quite naughty. I'm very disappointed in you today." Conflict resolution with a thrill! Or perhaps—just perhaps—you've discovered that there is a wider array of sensations that your body finds exciting. It doesn't have to be painful to be kinky. And you don't have to call it kinky for it to be something that elevates and enhances your vanilla.

As I said in the introduction, I love to hand my clients a dessert cookbook and challenge them to find the recipes that don't contain vanilla. Whether the goal is a simple sugar cookie or a richly layered German chocolate cake, we begin with the foundational element that brings every other ingredient together. In sex as in baking, vanilla is the starting point from which we add in all those lovely things that are enhanced and elevated by its presence: sprinkles of transparency, curiosity, openness, communication, passion, and always love.

Acknowledgments

Thank you so much to . . .

My agent, Jessica Alvarez, who understood my vision for *Sprinkles* from the very beginning. Your expertise and guidance have been invaluable.

Haven Iverson, who saw the potential in this project and immediately recognized who my readers were and why they needed this book.

Sarah Stanton, the editor who helped me craft its final form.

Frank Mons, for excising all my errant em dashes with surgical precision.

Tzipporah Horowitz and Lota Erinne, many thanks for your sensitivity and expert guidance.

My rabbis: Mark Miller and Megan Brudney, and my entire religious community for their unflagging acceptance of and encouragement for my work and my practice. Your love and support humble me.

As well as so many of my friends and colleagues who offered suggestions, readings, and support along the way, particularly Matt and Kellie Butler, Renee Graham, Elyssa Helfer, Faith Halverson-Ramos, Amy Marschall, Eric Morris, Ashley Perkins, Amy Saborsky, Erin Shapiro, Teisha Turner, Sabrina Valente, and Gillian Woldorf.

Notes

INTRODUCTION: I PROMISE, I'M NOT A PERVERT

1. Emma L. Turley, Nigel King, and Surya Monro, "'You Want to Be Swept Up in It All' Illuminating the Erotic in BDSM," *Psychology & Sexuality* 9, no. 2 (2018): 148–60.

2. Stefani Goerlich, *The Leather Couch: Clinical Practice with Kinky Clients* (New York: Routledge Press, 2020).

3. Marie Haaland, "Most People Hide Their Kinks Because They're Afraid Their Partner Will Leave," *New York Post*, June 9, 2020, nypost.com/2020/06/09/a-lot-of-people-hide-their-kinks-because -theyre-afraid-their-partner-will-leave-them/.

4. Debby Herbenick, Jessmyn Bowling, Tsung-Chieh (Jane) Fu, Brian Dodge, Lucia Guerra-Reyes, and Stephanie Sanders, "Sexual Diversity in the United States: Results from a Nationally Representative Probability Sample of Adult Women and Men," *PLoS ONE* 12, no. 7 (2017): 1–23, e0181198, doi.org/10.1371/journal .pone.0181198.

5. Herbenick et al., "Sexual Diversity in the United States."

6. Nele De Neef, Violette Coppens, Wim Huys, and Manuel Morrens, "Bondage-Discipline, Dominance-Submission, and Sadomasochism (BDSM) from an Integrative Biopsychosocial Perspective: A Systemic Review," *Sexual Medicine* 7, no. 129 (2020): 129–45.

7. Jillian Keenan, *Sex with Shakespeare: Here's Much to Do with Pain, but More with Love* (New York: William Morrow, 2017).

8. Christian C. Joyal and Julie Carpentier, "The Prevalence of Paraphilic Interests and Behavior in the General Population: A Provincial Survey," *Journal of Sex Research* 54, no. 2 (2017): 161–71, doi.org/10.1080/00224499.2016.1139034.

9. Joyal and Carpentier, "Prevalence of Paraphilic Interests."

10. Stephanie Tellier, "Advancing the Discourse: Disability and BDSM," *Sexuality and Disability* 35, no. 4, (2017): 485–93.

11. Brad J. Sagarin, Bert Cutler, Nadine Cutler, Kimberly A. Lawler-Sagarin, and Leslie Matuszewich, "Hormonal Changes and Couple Bonding in Consensual Sadomasochistic Activity," *Archives of Sexual Behavior* 38, no. 2 (2009): 186–200.

12. Roy F. Baumeister, "Masochism as Escape from Self," *Journal of Sex Research* 25, no. 1 (1988): 28–59.

13. Amity Pierce Buxton, "Paths and Pitfalls: How Heterosexual Spouses Cope When Their Husbands or Wives Come Out," *Journal of Couple & Relationship Therapy* 3, nos. 2–3 (2008): 95–109.

CHAPTER 1: NAVIGATING DISCOVERY AND DISCLOSURE

1. Jenn Sinrich, "The Truth about Keeping Secrets from Your Significant Other," MarthaStewart.com, September 11, 2018, marthastewart.com /7961562/truth-about-keeping-secret-from-your-significant-other.

2. Annette Kämmerer, "The Scientific Underpinnings and Impacts of Shame," Scientific American, August 9, 2019, scientificamerican .com/article/the-scientific-underpinnings-and-impacts-of-shame/.

3. Donna "Ara" Munier, "Neuroception 101: How the Mindbody Scans and Adapts for Safety and Danger," Neuroclastic.com, August 5, 2021, neuroclastic.com/neuroception-101-how-the-mindbody -scans-and-adapts-for-safety-and-danger/.

4. "What Does Fear Do to Our Vision?," *British Psychological Society Research Digest*, January 14, 2016, bps.org.uk/research-digest/what -does-fear-do-our-vision.

5. "Impact of Fear and Anxiety, Taking Charge of Your Health & Wellbeing," University of Minnesota (website), accessed December 18, 2021, takingcharge.csh.umn.edu/impact-fear-and-anxiety.

6. Eric Anderson, *The Monogamy Gap: Men, Love, and the Reality of Cheating* (New York: Oxford University Press, 2012).

7. Oz here means Australia.

8. "A Survey Reveals That 63% of BDSM Enthusiasts Have Cheated in a Committed Relationship with a BDSM Partner," Cision PR Newswire, August 9, 2021, prnewswire.com/news-releases/a-survey -reveals-that-63-of-bdsm-enthusiasts-have-cheated-in-a-committed -relationship-with-a-bdsm-partner-301351078.html.

9. "Survey Reveals That 63% of BDSM Enthusiasts Have Cheated in a Committed Relationship with a BDSM Partner."

10. Anderson, *Monogamy Gap*.

11. Bernadette Nathania Octaviana and Juneman Abraham, "Tolerance for Emotional Internet Infidelity and Its Correlate with Relationship Flourishing," *International Journal of Electrical and Computer Engineering (IJECE)* 8, no. 5 (October 2018): 3158–68.

12. "Financial Infidelity as Harmful as Sexual Infidelity in Married Life," Indo Asian News Service, December 12, 2019, indiatvnews .com/lifestyle/relationships-financial-infidelity-as-harmful-as-sexual -infidelity-in-married-life-571066.

13. "Financial Infidelity as Harmful as Sexual Infidelity in Married Life."

14. Dulcinea Pitagora, "Intimate Partner Violence in Sadomasochistic Relationships," *Sexual and Relationship Therapy* 31, no. 1 (2015): 95–108.

15. Anne O. Nomis, "The History of SSC (Safe Sane Consensual) vs. RACK (Risk-Aware Consensual Kink)," *History of the Dominatrix* (blog), February 8, 2018, historyofthedominatrix.com/blogs/blog /the-history-bdsm-consent-ssc-vs-rack.

16. "Road Safety Facts," Association for Safe International Road Travel, accessed December 12, 2021, asirt.org/safe-travel/road-safety-facts/.

17. Andrea Schmitz and Benji Jones, "Where the 11 Deadliest Animals in the US Live," Business Insider, September 8, 2021, businessinsider.com/deadliest-animals-us-dont-include-sharks -crocodiles-dogs-cows-2019-8.

18. D. J. Williams, Jeremy N. Thomas, Emily Prior, and M. Candace Christensen, "From 'SSC' and 'RACK' to the '4Cs': Introducing a New Framework for Negotiating BDSM Participation," *Electronic Journal of Human Sexuality* 17 (2014): 1–11.

19. *Scene* is the term used within BDSM to describe a specific BDSM experience. The scene may or may not be a sexual encounter, and what will or will not happen (and with whom) is negotiated by the partners before it begins.

20. Dan B. Allender and Tremper Longman III, *God Loves Sex: An Honest Conversation about Sexual Desire and Holiness* (Ada, MI: Baker Books, 2014).

21. William R. Stayton, *Sinless Sex: A Challenge to Religions* (Eugene, OR: Luminare Press, 2020).

CHAPTER 2: MEET YOUR KINKSTER!

1. David DePierre, *A Brief History of Oral Sex* (Jefferson, NC: Exposit Books, 2017).

2. Niklaus Largier, *In Praise of the Whip: A Cultural History of Arousal* (Brooklyn, NY: Zone Books, 2007).

3. Stefani Goerlich, *The Leather Couch: Clinical Practice with Kinky Clients* (New York: Routledge Press, 2020).

4. Julie Peakman, *The Pleasure's All Mine: A History of Perverse Sex* (London: Reaktion Books, 2013).

5. L. J. Charleston, "The Brutal Anti-masturbation Devices of the Victorian Era," *New Zealand Herald*, July 20, 2019, nzherald.co.nz /lifestyle/the-brutal-anti-masturbation-devices-of-the-victorian-era /BA3ABBTE2RP3LBY7BOEKHYKVMI/.

6. Elizabeth Sheehan, "Victorian Clitoridectomy: Isaac Baker Brown and His Harmless Operative Procedure," *Medical Anthropology Newsletter* 12, no. 4 (1981): 9–15.

7. "The Surprising History of Mental Illness Treatment," Baton Rouge Behavioral Health, January 13, 2021, batonrougebehavioral.com/the -surprising-history-of-mental-illness-treatment/.

8. Peakman, *Pleasure's All Mine*.

9. American Psychiatric Association, *Diagnostic and Statistical Manual of Mental Disorders*, 5th ed. (Washington, DC: American Psychological Association, 2013).

10. Juliet Richters, Richard O. De Visser, Chris E. Rissel, Andrew E. Grulich, and Anthony M. A. Smith, "Demographic and Psychosocial Features of Participants in Bondage and Discipline, 'Sadomasochism' or Dominance and Submission (BDSM): Data from a National Survey," *Journal of Sexual Medicine* 5, no. 7 (2008): 1660–68.

11. R. A. Sprott and A. Randall, "Health Disparities and Kink as an Unrecognized Sexual Minority," TASHRA 2016 Kink Health Survey Findings, Tashra: The Alternative Sexualities Health Research Alliance, November 2020, tashra.org/resources/health-disparities -and-kink-as-an-unrecognized-sexual-minority-why-it-matters-to -sexual-health-medicine/.

12. Michael P. Dentato, "The Minority Stress Perspective," American Psychological Association, April 2012, apa.org/pi/aids/resources /exchange/2012/04/minority-stress.

13. Richard A. Sprott and Anna M. Randall, *The Health and Healthcare Experiences of Kink-Oriented People: 2016 Survey Results*, TASHRA .org, November 19, 2016, 12d9eeb8-ede0-29a7-47b5-fe8d7e9e5513 .filesusr.com/ugd/115953_fdad42bb3879438080286975171a4aff.pdf.

14. Elyssa Helfer, "Strengths of Kink-Identified Clients," interview by Stefani Goerlich, January 13, 2022.

15. Goerlich, *Leather Couch*.

16. Ali Hébert and Angela Weaver, "An Examination of Personality Characteristics Associated with BDSM Orientations," *Canadian Journal of Human Sexuality* 23, no. 2 (2014): 106–15.

17. Sprott and Randall, *Health and Healthcare Experiences of Kink-Oriented People*.

18. Leigh Cowart, *Hurts So Good: The Science and Culture of Pain on Purpose* (New York: PublicAffairs, 2021).

19. Mary Kekatos, "Fifty Shades of HEALTH: Four Surprising Benefits of Kinky Sex," DailyMail.com, February 13, 2017, dailymail.co.uk/health /article-4220014/50-shades-HEALTH-surprising-benefits-kinky-sex.html.

20. Emma Sheppard, "Chronic Pain as Fluid, BDSM as Control," *Disability Studies Quarterly* 39, no. 2 (May 2019), doi.org/10.18061 /dsq.v39i2.6353.

21. Emma L. Turley, "Like Nothing I've Ever Felt Before: Understanding Consensual BDSM as Embodied Experience," *Psychology & Sexuality* 7, no. 2 (2016): 149–62.

22. Turley, "Like Nothing I've Ever Felt Before."

23. Brad Sagarin, Bert Cutler, Nadine Cutler, Kimberly Lawler-Sagarin, and Leslie Matuszewich, "Hormonal Changes and Couple Bonding in Consensual Sadomasochistic Activity," *Archives of Sexual Behavior* 38, no. 2 (2009): 186–200.

24. Kekatos, "Fifty Shades of HEALTH."

25. James K. Ambler, Ellen Lee, Kathryn Rebecca Klement, Tonio Loewald, Evelyn Comber, Sarah A. Hanson, Bert Cutler, Nadine Cutler, and Brad Sagarin, "Consensual BDSM Facilitates Role-Specific Altered States of Consciousness: A Preliminary Study," *Psychology of Consciousness Theory* 4, no. 1 (2017): 75–91.

26. Crystal Mundy and Jan D. Cioe, "Exploring the Relationship Between Paraphilic Interests, Sex, and Sexual and Life Satisfaction in Non-Clinical Samples," *Canadian Journal of Human Sexuality* 28, no. 3 (2019): 304–16.

27. Turley, "Like Nothing I've Ever Felt Before."

28. Ali Hébert and Angela Weaver, "Perks, Problems, and the People Who Play: A Qualitative Exploration of Dominant and Submissive BDSM Roles," *Canadian Journal of Human Sexuality* 24, no. 1 (April 2015): 49–62.

29. Cassandra Damm, Michael P. Dentato, and Nikki Busch, "Unravelling Intersecting Identities: Understanding the Lives of People Who Practice BDSM," *Psychology and Sexuality* 9, no. 1 (December 2017): 1–17.

30. Damm, Dentato, and Busch, "Unravelling Intersecting Identities."

31. Roy F. Baumeister, "Masochism as Escape from Self," *Journal of Sex Research* 25, no. 1 (1988): 28–59.

32. Baumeister, "Masochism as Escape from Self."

33. Hébert and Weaver, "Perks, Problems, and the People Who Play."

34. Hébert and Weaver.

35. Hébert and Weaver.

36. Katherine Martinez, "Somebody's Fetish: Self-Objectification and Body Satisfaction among Consensual Sadomasochists," *Journal of Sex Research* 53, no. 1 (2016): 35–44.

37. Turley, "Like Nothing I've Ever Felt Before," 149–62.

38. Mundy and Cioe, "Exploring the Relationship Between Paraphilic Interests."

39. Corie Hammers, "Corporeality, Sadomasochism and Sexual Trauma," *Body & Society* 20, no. 2 (2014): 69–90.

40. Damm, Dentato, and Busch, "Unravelling Intersecting Identities."

41. Hébert and Weaver, "Perks, Problems, and the People Who Play."

42. Hébert and Weaver.

43. Hébert and Weaver.

44. Brad J. Sagarin, Bert Cutler, Nadine Cutler, Kimberly A. Lawler-Sagarin, and Leslie Matuszewich, "Hormonal Changes and Couple Bonding in Consensual Sadomasochistic Activity," *Archives of Sexual Behavior* 38 no. 2 (2008): 186–200, doi.org/10.1007/s10508-008-9374-5.

45. Sagarin et al., "Hormonal Changes and Couple Bonding in Consensual Sadomasochistic Activity."

46. Peggy J. Kleinplatz, "Learning from Extraordinary Lovers: Lessons from the Edge," in *Sadomasochism: Powerful Pleasures,* ed. Peggy J. Kleinplatz and Charles Moser (Binghamton, NY: Haworth Press, 2006), 325–48.

47. Kleinplatz, "Learning from Extraordinary Lovers."

48. Kate Hakala, "There's a Big Benefit to BDSM That Nobody's Talking About," Mic.com, February 10, 2015, mic.com/articles/110294/there-s-a-positive-benefit-to-bdsm-everyone-s-been-overlooking.

49. Cowart, *Hurts So Good.*

CHAPTER 3: FEELING VANILLA IN A THIRTY-ONE-FLAVORS KIND OF WORLD

1. Michael Slepian, "The Problem with Keeping a Secret," Society for Personality and Social Psychology, July 1, 2019, spsp.org/news-center/blog/arvard-keeping-secrets.

2. Kirsten Weir, "Exposing the Hidden World of Secrets," *Monitor on Psychology* 51, no. 6 (2020): 74.

3. Weir, "Exposing the Hidden World of Secrets"

4. Eric W. Dolan, "New Psychology Research Sheds Light on How the

Experience of Keeping a Secret Is Affected by Relationship Quality," PsyPost, August 7, 2021, psypost.org/2021/08/new-psychology -research-sheds-light-on-how-the-experience-of-keeping-a-secret-is -affected-relationship-quality-61650.

5. Mariela E. Jaffe and Maria Douneva, "Secretive and Close? How Sharing Secrets May Impact Perceptions of Distance," *PLoS One* 15, no. 6 (2020), doi.org/10.1371/journal.pone.0233953.

6. Tara M. Busch, "Perceived Acceptability of Sexual and Romantic Fantasizing," *Sexuality & Culture* 24 (2020): 848–62.

7. Barry McCarthy, MSTI lecture 2020.

8. Busch, "Perceived Acceptability of Sexual and Romantic Fantasizing."

9. "Key Statistics from the National Survey of Family Growth—N Listing," Centers for Disease Control and Prevention, National Center for Health Statistics, July 17, 2017, cdc.gov/nchs/nsfg/key _statistics/n.htm#numberlifetime.

10. Justin Lehmiller, *Tell Me What You Want* (New York: Hachette Go, 2018).

11. Roy F. Baumeister, "Masochism as Escape from Self," *Journal of Sex Research* 25, no. 1 (1988): 28–59.

12. Debra W. Soh, "1 in 6 People Has a Sex Fetish. A Neuroscientist Explains Why," *Men's Health*, May 13, 2016, menshealth.com/sex -women/a19520718/extreme-fetishes/.

13. Julia Simner, James E. A. Hughes, and Noam Sagiv, "Objectum Sexuality: A Sexual Orientation Linked with Autism and Synaesthesia," *Scientific Reports* 9, no. 19874 (2019), doi.org/10 .1038/s41598-019-56449-0.

14. Genki Ferguson, "Objectophilia: On the People Who Fall in Love with Inanimate Things," Literary Hub, April 30, 2021, lithub.com /objectophilia-on-the-people-who-fall-in-love-with-inanimate-things/.

15. Brynn Tannehill, *Everything You Ever Wanted to Know about Trans (But Were Afraid to Ask)* (Philadelphia, PA: Jessica Kingsley, 2019).

16. Sari Reisner, Tonia Poteat, JoAnne Keatley, Mauro Cabral, Tampose Mothopeng, Emilia Dunham, Claire E. Holland, Ryan Max, and Stefan D. Baral, "Global Health Burden and Needs of Transgender Populations: A Review," *Lancet* 388, no. 10042 (2019): 412–36.

17. Lehmiller, *Tell Me What You Want*.

18. Lehmiller.

19. Brett Kahr, *Who's Been Sleeping In Your Head? The Secret World of Sexual Fantasies* (New York: Basic Books, 2009).

20. Justin Lehmiller, "Seven Fascinating Facts about Sexual Fantasies," Sex & Psychology, May 15, 2015, sexandpyschology.com/blog/2015 /5/15/seven-fascinating-facts-about-sexual-fantasies.

21. "The Kinsey Scale," Kinsey Institute, accessed January 28, 2022, kinseyinstitute.org/research/publications/kinsey-scale.php.

22. Jill L. Kays and Mark A. Yarhouse, "Resilient Factors in Mixed Orientation Couples: Current State of the Research," *American Journal of Family Therapy* 38, no. 4 (2010): 334–43.

23. Baumeister, "Masochism as Escape from Self."

24. Kendra Cherry, "What Are the Jungian Archetypes?" Verywell Mind, last updated December 16, 2022, verywellmind.com/what-are-jungs -4-major-archetypes-2795439.

25. Chelsea Wakefield, "In Search of Aphrodite: Working with Archetypes and an Inner Cast of Characters in Women with Low Sexual Desire," *Sexual and Relationship Therapy* 29, no. 1 (2014): 31–41.

26. Wakefield, "In Search of Aphrodite."

27. Christopher N. Cascio, Matthew Brook O'Donnell, Francis J. Tinney, Matthew Lieberman, Shelley Taylor, Victor Strecher, and Emily Falk, "Self-Affirmation Activates Brain Systems Associated with Self-Related Processing and Reward and Is Reinforced by Future Orientation," *Social Cognitive and Affective Neuroscience* 11, no. 4 (2015): 621–29; Emily

Falk, Matthew Brook O'Donnell, Christopher N. Cascio, Francis Tinney, Yoona Kang, Matthew Lieberman, Shelley Taylor, Lawrence An, Ken Resnicow, and Victor Strecher, "Self-Affirmation Alters the Brain's Response to Health Messages and Subsequent Behavior Change," *Proceedings of the National Academy of Sciences* 112, no. 7 (2015): 1977–82; Catherine Moore, "Positive Daily Affirmations: Is There Science Behind It?" PositivePsychology.com, March 4, 2019, positivepsychology .com/daily-affirmations/.

28. "The Power of the Placebo Effect," Harvard Health Publishing, December 13, 2021, health.harvard.edu/mental-health/the-power-of -the-placebo-effect.

29. Madeleine M. Castellanos, *Wanting to Want: What Kills Your Sex Life and How to Keep It Alive* (New York: Tao Health, 2014).

30. Laurie Mintz, *Becoming Cliterate: Why Orgasm Equality Matters— and How to Get It* (San Francisco, CA: HarperOne, 2017).

31. Mintz, *Becoming Cliterate*.

32. Castellanos, *Wanting to Want*.

33. Eric W. Dolan, "Good, Giving, and Game: Research Confirms That Dan Savage's Sex Advice Works," PsyPost, October 25, 2014, psypost.org/2014/10/good-giving-game-research-confirms-dan -savages-sex-advice-works-28965.

34. Arthur Stamps, "Visual Permeability, Locomotive Permeability, Safety, and Enclosure," *Environment and Behavior* 37, no. 5 (2005): 587–619.

CHAPTER 4: FINDING YOUR SPRINKLES

1. K. W. Colyard, "Who Reads Romance Novels? Infographic Tells All," Bustle, June 14, 2016, bustle.com/articles/166802-who-reads -romance-novels-this-infographic-has-the-answer.

2. Justin Lehmiller, "The 7 Most Common Sex Fantasies—And How Many People Have Ever Had Them," Sex and Psychology, March 13,

2019, sexandpsychology.com/blog/2019/3/13/the-7-most-common
-sex-fantasies-and-how-many-people-have-ever-had-them/.

3. Michael Harris, "Let Your Mind Wander," *Discover* 38, no. 5 (June 2017).

4. Anna Clemens, "When the Mind's Eye Is Blind," *Scientific American*,
August 1, 2018, scientificamerican.com/article/when-the-minds-eye
-is-blind1/.

5. Laurie Mintz, *Becoming Cliterate: Why Orgasm Equality Matters—
and How to Get It* (San Francisco, CA: HarperOne, 2017).

6. Berakhot 62a:4, William Davidson Talmud, Sefaria, accessed February
10, 2022, sefaria.org/Berakhot.62a.4?lang=bi&with=all&lang2=bi.

7. Marty Klein, *His Porn, Her Pain: Confronting American's Porn Panic
with Honest Talk about Sex* (Santa Barbara, CA: Praeger, 2016).

8. Markham Heid, "How Hot Women Help You Destress," *Men's
Health*, July 10, 2013, menshealth.com/health/a19544656/how-hot
-women-help-you-de-stress/.

9. E. J. Dickson, Kristen Hubby, and Nico Lang, "11 Unexpected
Benefits of Watching Porn," DailyDot, July 16, 2020, dailydot.com
/nsfw/guides/porn-benefits/.

10. Nicole Prause and James G. Pfaus, "Viewing Sexual Stimuli Associated
with Greater Sexual Responsiveness, Not Erectile Dysfunction,"
Sexual Medicine 3, no. 2 (2015), doi.org/10.1002/sm2.58.

11. Mark McCormack and Liam Wignall, "Enjoyment, Exploration and
Education: Understanding the Consumption of Pornography among
Young Men with Non-Exclusive Sexual Orientations," *Sociology* 51, no.
5 (2017): 975–91.

12. Anna Pulley, "9 Surprising Reasons Why You Should Be Watching
Porn," Salon, September 2, 2017, salon.com/2017/09/02/9
-surprising-reasons-why-you-should-be-watching-porn_partner/.

13. Candida Royalle, "Pornography Can Be Good for Consumers," *New*

York Times, November 11, 2012, nytimes.com/roomfordebate/2012
/11/11/does-pornography-deserve-its-bad-rap/pornography-can-be
-good-for-consumers#:~:text=It%20can%20give%20you%20ideas,or
%20disgust%20you%20at%20worst.

14. Steph Auteri, "The History of Sensate Focus, and How We Self-
Educate When It Comes to Evolving Therapeutic Techniques,"
AASECT, May 2014, aasect.org/history-sensate-focus-and-how-we
-self-educate-when-it-comes-evolving-therapeutic-techniques.

CHAPTER 5: TASTE-TESTING OTHER FLAVORS

1. C. S. Lewis, *Mere Christianity* (New York: Macmillan, 1977).

2. "Science Says This Is How Many Dates You Have to Go On Before
You Find 'The One,'" Her, accessed February 19, 2022, her.ie/life
/whats-your-number-study-finds-the-average-number-of-dates-and
-relationships-before-we-find-the-one-90330#:~:text=The%20biggest
%20difference%20between%20men,while%20women%20will
%20have%20five.

3. Stefani Goerlich, *Kink-Affirming Practice: Culturally Competent
Therapy from the Leather Chair* (New York: Routledge, 2022).

4. Jack Morin, *The Erotic Mind: Unlocking the Inner Sources of Passion
and Fulfillment* (New York: Harper Perennial, 1996).

5. Hannah M. E. Rogak and Jennifer Jo Connor, "Practice of
Consensual BDSM and Relationship Satisfaction," *Sexual and
Relationship Therapy* 33, no. 4 (2018): 454–69.

6. Morin, *Erotic Mind*, 76.

7. Bat Sheva Marcus, "The Ultimate Sex Book Club Entry," Facebook,
March 18, 2022, 2:33 pm.

8. "Predicament Play, Foundation for Sex Positive Culture," September
19, 2017, thefspc.org/event/predicament-play/.

9. Princess Kali, *Enough to Make You Blush: Exploring Erotic Humiliation* (San Jose, CA: Erotication, 2015).

CHAPTER 6: WHAT'S NORMAL, ANYWAY?

1. "FAQs and Sex Information," Kinsey Institute, accessed May 26, 2022, kinseyinstitute.org/research/faq.php.

2. "FAQs and Sex Information."

3. Dena Bunis, "Two-Thirds of Older Adults Are Interested in Sex, Poll Says," AARP, May 3, 2018, aarp.org/health/healthy-living/info-2018 /older-sex-sexual-health-survey.html.

4. "Let's Talk about Sex," National Poll on Healthy Aging, Institute on Healthcare Policy and Innovation, University of Michigan, May 3, 2018, healthyagingpoll.org/reports-more/report/lets-talk-about-sex.

5. Anna Rahmanan, "Study Reveals Average Amount of Sex People Are Having at Your Age," TimeOut.com, August 28, 2017, timeout.com /usa/blog/study-reveals-average-amount-of-sex-people-are-having -at-your-age-082817#:~:text=Specifically%2C%20the%20team %20behind%20the,or%2086%20times%20per%20year).

6. Debby Herbenick, Michael Reece, Vanessa Schick, Stephanie A. Sanders, Brian Dodge, and J. Dennis Fortenberry, "Sexual Behavior in the United States: Results from a National Probability Sample of Men and Women Ages 14–94," *Journal of Sexual Medicine* 7, no. S5 (2010): 255–65.

7. Mona Chalabi, "Dear Mona, I Masturbate More Than Once a Day. Am I Normal?" fivethirtyeight.com, May 30, 2014, fivethirtyeight.com /features/dear-mona-i-masturbate-more-than-once-a-day-am-i-normal/.

8. Herbernick et al., "Sexual Behavior in the United States."

9. Herbernick et al.

10. Peter Ueda, Catherine Mercer, Cyrus Ghaznavi, and Debby Herbenick, "Trends in Frequency of Sexual Activity and Numbers

of Sexual Partners among Adults 18 to 44 Years in the US, 2000–2018," *JAMA Network Open* 3, no. 6 (2020), doi.org/10.1001/jamanetworkopen.2020.3833.

11. Austin Institute for the Study of Family and Culture, "How Often Do American's Have Sex?" relationshipsinamerica.com, 2014, thepublicdiscourse.com/2014/12/14131/.

12. Arthur Zuckerman, "50 Cheating Statistics: 2020/2021 Demographics, Reasons & Who Cheats More," CompareCamp.com, May 29, 2020, comparecamp.com/cheating-statistics/.

13. Wendy Wang, "Who Cheats More? The Demographics of Infidelity in America," Institute for Family Studies, January 10, 2018, ifstudies.org/blog/who-cheats-more-the-demographics-of-cheating-in-america.

14. "Cheating Spouse Survey Results," Truth about Deception, accessed May 26, 2022, truthaboutdeception.com/community-features/online-quizzes/cheating-spouse-results.html.

15. "Cheating Spouse Survey Results."

16. "Infidelity: The Cold Hard Truth about Cheating," LA Intelligence, March 10, 2021, laintelligence.com/infidelity-the-cold-hard-truth-about-cheating/.

17. Justin Lehmiller, "How Similar or Different Are the Sex Lives of Gay and Straight Men?" Sex & Psychology, June 28, 2021, sexandpsychology.com/blog/2021/6/28/how-similar-or-different-are-the-sex-lives-of-gay-and-straight-men/.

18. David A. Frederick, Brian Joseph Gillespie, Janet Lever, Vincent Berardi, and Justin R. Garcia, "Debunking Lesbian Bed Death: Using Coarsened Exact Matching to Compare Sexual Practices and Satisfaction of Lesbian and Heterosexual Women," *Archives of Sexual Behavior* 50, no. 8 (November 2021): 3601–19, doi.org/10.1007/s10508-021-02096-4.

19. Megan Martin, "Debunking the 'Lesbian Bed Death' Myth," Dame, March 12, 2021, dame.com/do-lesbians-have-less-sex/.

20. Frederick et al., "Debunking Lesbian Bed Death."

21. Mary Brain, "How Often Do Gay Couples Have Sex?" William Russell for Congress, March 21, 2019, williamrussellforcongress .com/how-often-do-gay-couples-have-sex/.

22. "National Survey of Sexual Health and Behavior," Indiana University Bloomington, accessed May 26, 2022, nationalsexstudy.indiana.edu /keyfindings/index.html.

23. Hannah Roberts, Angus Clark, Carter Sherman, Mary M. Heitzig, and Brian M. Hicks, "Age, Sex, and Other Demographic Trends in Sexual Behavior in the United States: Initial Findings of the Sexual Behaviors, Internet Use, and Psychological Adjustment Survey," *PLoS One* 16, no. 8 (2021), doi.org/10.1371/journal.pone.0255371.

24. "General FAQ," Asexual Visibility and Education Network, accessed May 26, 2022, asexuality.org/?q=general.html#ex2.

25. Morag A. Yule, Lori A., Brotto, and Boris B. Gorzalka, "Sexual Fantasy and Masturbation among Asexual Individuals," *Canadian Journal of Human Sexuality* 23, no. 2 (2014): 89–95, utpjournals .press/doi/abs/10.3138/cjhs.2409.

26. Angela Chen, *Ace: What Asexuality Reveals about Desire, Society, and the Meaning of Sex* (Boston: Beacon Press, 2021).

27. Laurie Mintz, *Becoming Cliterate: Why Orgasm Equality Matters—and How to Get It* (New York: HarperOne, 2017).

28. Laurie Mintz, "The Orgasm Gap: Facts Behind Male vs Female Orgasm & Sexual Solutions," drlauriemintz.com, last updated November 26, 2019, drlauriemintz.com/post/the-orgasm-gap-facts -behind-male-vs-female-orgasm-sexual-solutions.

29. Mintz, "The Orgasm Gap."

30. Dana Lising, "Differences Between Penis and Clitoris," Tantra-Lising, April 29, 2014, tantralising.co.uk/blog/article/differences -between-penis-and-clitoris/.

31. Michelle Spoto, "The Biology of the Orgasm," Reporter, May 3, 2014, reporter.rit.edu/features/biology-orgasm.

32. Sophia Mitrokostas, "Here's What Happens to Your Body and Brain When You Orgasm," ScienceAlert, January 26, 2019, sciencealert .com/here-s-what-happens-to-your-brain-when-you-orgasm.

33. Mitrokostas, "Here's What Happens to Your Body and Brain When You Orgasm."

34. Katie Smith, "This Is What Happens to Your Brain after Sex," Insider, June 28, 2018, businessinsider.com/what-happens-to-your -brain-after-sex-2018-6.

35. C. Y. Hsu, C. L. Lin, and C. H. Kao, "Irritable Bowel Syndrome Is Associated Not Only with Organic but Also Psychogenic Erectile Dysfunction," *International Journal of Impotence Research* 27, no. 6 (November–December 2015): 233–38, doi.org/10.1038/ijir.2015.25.

36. Emma Sheppard, "Chronic Pain as Fluid, BDSM as Control," *Disability Studies Quarterly* 39, no. 2 (2019), doi.org/10.18061/dsq .v39i2.6353.

37. Ruth Cohn, *Coming Home to Passion: Restoring Loving Sexuality in Couples with Histories of Childhood Trauma and Neglect* (Santa Barbara, CA: ABC-Clio/Praeger, 2011).

CHAPTER 7: WHAT DOES "NORMAL" KINK LOOK LIKE?

1. "Welcome to Fetlife," FetLife, accessed June 1, 2022, https://fetlife.com/.

2. Midori, "Midori's Negotiations Technique," interview by Stefani Goerlich, April 19, 2022.

3. Stefani Goerlich, *The Leather Couch: Clinical Practice with Kinky Clients* (New York: Routledge Press, 2020).

4. Larry Solomon, "A Christian Husband's Guide to Grooming His Young Wife," accessed June 1, 2022, biblicalgenderroles.com/a -christian-husbands-guide-to-grooming-his-young-wife/.

5. Solomon, "A Christian Husband's Guide to Grooming His Young Wife."

6. Adriana Grimes, "The Science of Fetishes," *Osmosis Magazine*, no. 1 (2019), scholarship.richmond.edu/osmosis/vol2019/iss1/5.

7. Debra W. Soh, "1 in 6 People Has a Sex Fetish—Here Are a Few of the Craziest," *Women's Health*, June 7, 2016, womenshealthmag.com /sex-and-love/a19976035/extreme-fetishes-0/.

8. Sarah Kramer, "Here's How Common 'Abnormal' Sexual Fetishes Actually Are," Insider, March 22, 2016, businessinsider.com /common-sexual-fetishes-abnormal-normal-kink-2016-3#:~: text=While%20only%20a%20quarter%20of,had%20actually %20engaged%20in%20voyeurism.

9. Kramer, "Here's How Common 'Abnormal' Sexual Fetishes Actually Are."

10. Grimes, "The Science of Fetishes."

11. Claudia Scorolli, Stefano Ghirlanda, Magnus Enquist, S. Zattoni, and Emmanuele A. Janini, "Relative Prevalence of Different Fetishes," *Journal of Impotence Research* 19, no. 4 (February 2017): 432–37.

12. Grimes, "The Science of Fetishes."

13. "The Cost of Coming Out: LGBT Youth Homelessness," Lesley University, accessed June 1, 2022, lesley.edu/article/the-cost-of -coming-out-lgbt-youth-homelessness.

14. "Polyamorous and Leather Families," House of Decorum, accessed June 1, 2022, houseofdecorum.org/workshops-classes/polyamorous -leather-families/.

15. Douglas Kenrick, Vladus Griskevicius, Steven Neuberg, and Mark Schaller, "Renovating the Pyramid of Needs: Contemporary Extensions Built Upon Ancient Foundations," *Perspectives on Psychological Science* 5, no. 3 (2010): 292–314.

CHAPTER 8: WHEN ONE FLAVOR ISN'T ENOUGH

1. Jennifer Rubin, Amy C. Moors, Jes L. Matsick, Ali Ziegler, and Terri Conley, "On the Margins: Considering Diversity among Consensually Non-monogamous Relationships," *Journal für Psychologie* 22, no. 1 (2014): 1–25.

2. Ethan Czuy Levine, Debby Herbenick, Omar Martinez, Tsung-Chieh Fu, and Brian Dodge, "Open Relationships, Nonconsensual Nonmonogamy, and Monogamy among U.S. Adults: Findings from the 2012 National Survey of Sexual Health and Behavior," *Archives of Sexual Behavior* 47, no. 5 (July 2018): 1439–50.

3. Nicki Lisa Cole, "What Is a Norm? Why Does It Matter?" ThoughtCo, August 27, 2018, thoughtco.com/why-a-norm-matter-3026644#:~:text=%22Normal%22%20refers%20to%20that%20which,of%20whether%20it%20actually%20is.

4. Claire Kimberley and Robert McGinley, "Changes in the Swinging Lifestyle: A US National and Historical Comparison," *Culture, Health & Sexuality* 21, no. 2 (2019): 219–32.

5. Andie Nordgren, "The Short Instructional Manifesto for Relationship Anarchy," Andie's Log, July 6, 2012, log.andie.se/post/26652940513/the-short-instructional-manifesto-for-relationship.

6. "What Is RA?" Relationship-Anarchy.com, accessed June 6, 2022, relationship-anarchy.com/about/.

7. Nick Levine, "What Is 'Radical Monogamy'?" Vice, March 8, 2022, vice.com/en/article/m7vxxy/what-is-radical-monogamy.

CHAPTER 9: WHEN IT ALL FEELS HOPELESS

1. "Divorce Rate by State 2022," World Population Review, accessed June 6, 2022, worldpopulationreview.com/state-rankings/divorce-rate-by-state.

2. Garrett Callahan, "Divorce and Religion: What Different Faiths Say about Ending a Marriage," DivorceNet, accessed June 6, 2022, divorcenet.com/resources/divorce-and-religion.html.

3. Shelby B. Scott, Galena K. Rhoades, Scott M. Stanley, Elizabeth S. Allen, and Howard Markman, "Reasons for Divorce and Recollections of Premarital Intervention: Implications for Improving Relationship Education," *Couple & Family Psychology* 2, no. 2 (2013): 131–45, doi.org/10.1037/a0032025.

4. Elizabeth Gilbert, *Eat, Pray, Love* (New York: Riverhead Books, 2007).

5. D. Ivan Young, *Break Up, Don't Break Down* (Houston: Reality-N-3D Publishing, 2010).

6. Martha Stark, "Transformation of Relentless Hope: A Relational Approach to Sadomasochism," Wild Apricot, accessed June 6, 2022, aps-tn.wildapricot.org/resources/Documents/Martha%20Stark%20 -%20Relentless%20Hope%20for%20APS.pdf.

7. Marty Klein and Charles Moser, "SM (Sadomasochistic) Interests as an Issue in a Child Custody Proceeding," *Journal of Homosexuality* 50, nos. 2–3 (2008): 233–42.

8. Wesley Fenza, "BDSM, Kink, and Child Custody," Fenza Legal Services, October 1, 2019, fenzalaw.com/blog-index/bdsm-kink-and -child-custody/.

9. Gabrielle Hartley and Elena Brower, *Better Apart: The Radically Positive Way to Separate* (New York: Harper Wave, 2021).

10. Joe Carter, "5 Facts about No-Fault Divorce," Ethics & Religious Liberty Commission, August 16, 2019, erlc.com/resource-library /articles/5-facts-about-no-fault-divorce/.

11. Paul R. Amato and Juliana M. Sobolewski, "The Effects of Divorce and Marital Discord on Adult Children's Psychological Well-Being," *American Sociological Review* 66, no. 6 (December 2001): 900–921.

12. Caitlin Halligan, I. Joyce Chang, and David Knox, "Positive Effects of Parental Divorce on Undergraduates," *Journal of Divorce & Remarriage* 55, no. 7 (2014): 557–67.

13. Paul R. Amato, "The Consequences of Divorce for Adults and Children: An Update," *Drustvena Istrazivanja; Zagreb* 23, no. 1 (2014), doi.org/10.5559/di.23.1.01.

14. Halligan, Chang, and Knox, "Positive Effects of Parental Divorce on Undergraduates."

15. Grant Mohi, "Positive Outcomes of Divorce: A Multi-Method Study on the Effects of Parental Divorce on Children" (honors thesis, University of Central Florida, 2014), stars.library.ucf.edu /honorstheses1990-2015/1601.

16. Mohi, "Positive Outcomes of Divorce."

17. Mohi.

18. Halligan, Chang, and Knox, "Positive Effects of Parental Divorce on Undergraduates."

19. Halligan, Chang, and Knox.

20. Rosemary Bernstein, "Parental Divorce and Romantic Attachment in Young Adulthood: Important Role of Problematic Beliefs," *Marriage & Family Review* 48, no. 8 (2012), doi.org/10.1080 /01494929.2012.700910.

CHAPTER 10: COCREATING THE FUTURE YOU WANT FOR YOURSELF (AND EACH OTHER)

1. Thomas H. Holmes and Robert H. Rahe, "The Social Readjustment Rating Scale," *Journal of Psychosomatic Research* 11, no. 2 (1967): 213–21.

2. Saul McLeod, "SRRS—Stress of Life Events," Simply Psychology, 2010, simplypsychology.org/SRRS.html.

3. Marvin S. Gerst, Igor Grant, Joel Yager, and Hervey Sweetwood, "The Reliability of the Social Readjustment Rating Scale: Moderate and Long-Term Stability," *Journal of Psychosomatic Research* 22, no. 6 (1978): 519–23.

4. "Social Readjustment Rating Scale," Brandeis University, accessed June 12, 2022, brandeis.edu/roybal/docs/Social%20Readjustment%20rating%20scale_Website.pdf.

5. Amy Muise and Emily A. Impett, "Good, Giving, and Game: The Relationship Benefits of Communal Sexual Motivation," *Social Psychology and Personality Science* 6, no. 2 (February 2014): 164–72, doi.org/10.1177/1948550614553641.

6. Reuma Gadassi, Lior Eadan Bar-Nahum, Sarah Newhouse, Ragnar Anderson, Julia R. Heiman, Eshkol Rafaeli, and Erick Janssen, "Perceived Partner Responsiveness Mediates the Association Between Sexual and Marital Satisfaction: A Daily Diary Study in Newlywed Couples," *Archives of Sexual Behavior* 45 (2016): 109–20.

7. Carolyn Birnie-Porter and Mitchell Hunt, "Does Relationship Status Matter for Sexual Satisfaction? The Roles of Intimacy and Attachment Avoidance in Sexual Satisfaction Across Five Types of Ongoing Sexual Relationships," *Canadian Journal of Human Sexuality* 24, no. 2 (2015): 174–83.

8. Jenna Marie Strizzi, Camilla Stine Øverup, Ana Ciprić, Gert Martin Hald, and Bente Træen, "BDSM: Does It Hurt or Help Sexual Satisfaction, Relationship Satisfaction, and Relationship Closeness?" *Journal of Sex Research* 59, no. 2 (2022): 248–57.

9. Muise and Impett, "Good, Giving, and Game."

10. Muise and Impett.

11. Gadassi et al., "Perceived Partner Responsiveness."

12. Sarah LaChance Adams, "Simone de Beauvoir and the Ethics of Seduction," Iai News, March 25, 2022, iai.tv/articles/simone-de-beauvoir-and-the-ethics-of-seduction-auid-2087.

13. LaChance Adams, "Simone de Beauvoir and the Ethics of Seduction."

14. Strizzi et al., "BDSM."

15. Chris Donaghue, *Sex Outside the Lines: Authentic Sexuality in a Sexually Dysfunctional Culture* (Dallas: BenBella Books, 2015).

16. Tammy Nelson, *Open Monogamy: A Guide to Co-creating Your Ideal Relationship Agreement* (Boulder, CO: Sounds True, 2021).

17. Author unknown.

Index

About the Author

Stefani Goerlich is an expert in working with gender, relationship, and sexually diverse folks as well as religious minorities and has dedicated her career to supporting clients who have had their bodies and their sexuality weaponized against them.

She earned a master's degree in social work from Wayne State University; completed her post-graduate certificate in sex therapy at the University of Michigan, where she is on the teaching faculty of the Sexual Health Certificate Program; and holds a PhD in clinical sexology, an emerging academic discipline focusing on sexuality research and treatment.

An AASECT-certified sex therapist and board-certified sexology diplomate licensed to practice in four states, Stefani lives with her husband and son in Detroit, Michigan, where she offers sex, relationship, and mental health therapy to members of the GSRD community, their partners, and their families. She is an active member of her religious community and spends her free time traveling, reading, and cross-stitching. She loves manatees, folk music, and anything pink or sparkly.

When it comes to her clinical philosophy, Stefani states that "my mission, first and foremost, is to help my clients build positive, happy, healthy relationships with their bodies, their partners, and themselves. I want them to see that sex and intimacy can be a positive force for good in their lives. That is what brings me to work every. single. day."

Stefani believes . . .

- Pleasure, intimacy, and connection are valid needs to have and to ethically pursue.

- People are entitled to define their sexuality on their own terms.

- No one should be judged or shamed for their sexual desires.

- We each have a moral and ethical obligation to seek out ethical, consensual ways to express our desires.

- Honest, accurate, and comprehensive sex education is a human right and necessary to give folks the knowledge and tools they need to have fulfilling, healthy, happy relationships.

- Most people are sexual beings and want to have meaningful sex lives with partners they trust, care about, and choose. This is true regardless of their gender, survivor status, disability, culture, or faith tradition.

- Folks who are asexual or sex averse are valid and entitled to respect.

- People should have agency and freedom in their sexual decision-making, including when, with whom, and under what conditions they have sex. This includes sex work.

- Sexuality and intimacy are sacred gifts, and sexual expression does not contradict religious belief.

- Each and every human being is born exactly as they are meant to be and no one has the right to force change upon another simply because they disagree.

Stefani does *not* believe . . .

- Everyone must have sex to be whole and healthy human beings.

- We have the right or the skill to change someone's sexual or gender identity.

- Sex has to be kinky, nonmonogamous, or pansexual in order to be good sex.

- Kink, nonmonogamy, or pansexuality are signs of mental illness.

- Accepting someone's sexuality means engaging in it with them, either visually, verbally, or physically.

- Sex is *always* positive, healthy, and good. (Sex can and is used in harmful ways.)

- Sex is a cure-all.

About Sounds True

Sounds True was founded in 1985 by Tami Simon with a clear mission: to disseminate spiritual wisdom. Since starting out as a project with one woman and her tape recorder, we have grown into a multimedia publishing company with a catalog of more than 3,000 titles by some of the leading teachers and visionaries of our time, and an ever-expanding family of beloved customers from across the world.

In more than three decades of evolution, Sounds True has maintained our focus on our overriding purpose and mission: to wake up the world. We offer books, audio programs, online learning experiences, and in-person events to support your personal growth and awakening, and to unlock our greatest human capacities to love and serve.

At SoundsTrue.com you'll find a wealth of resources to enrich your journey, including our weekly Insights at the Edge podcast, free downloads, and information about our nonprofit Sounds True Foundation, where we strive to remove financial barriers to the materials we publish through scholarships and donations worldwide.

To learn more, please visit SoundsTrue.com/freegifts or call us toll-free at 800.333.9185.

Together, we can wake up the world.

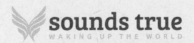